The CARB CYCLING DIET

The CARB CYCLING DIET

ROMAN MALKOV, MD

Optimize your health, lose weight, feel great—without giving up the foods you love

PHOTOS BY PETER FIELD PECK

HATHERLEIGH PRESS
New York • London

Hatherleigh Press
5-22 46th Avenue, Suite 200
Long Island City, NY 11101
www.hatherleighpress.com

Library of Congress Cataloging-in-Publication Data

Malkov, Roman, 1965–
  The carb cycling diet / Roman Malkov.
      p. cm.
  Includes bibliographical references.
  ISBN 978-1-57826-309-7
  1. Low-carbohydrate diet. I. Title.
  RM237.73.M35 2006
  613.2'83--dc22

                              2005031500

The Carb Cycling Diet is available for bulk purchase, special promotions, and premiums. For information on reselling and special purchase opportunities, call 1-800-528-2550 and ask for the Special Sales Manager.

Interior design by Deborah Miller and Jacinta Monniere
Cover design by Sarah Stern

10 9 8
Printed in the United States

I dedicate this book to my grandmother, Dina.

Acknowledgments

I would like to express my deepest thanks to everyone who has endured all the hard work on this book at Hatherleigh Press. I cannot imagine a better publishing company for my book. I am impressed by everyone's energy and enthusiasm in effort to deliver health and fitness messages out to the public.

Special thanks to Kevin and Andrea.

CONTENTS

Preface   13

PART 1 SCIENCE

CHAPTER 1:   Creating a Diet That Really Works:
The Proven Power of the Carb Cycling Diet   21

CHAPTER 2:   The Problem with Calorie Restricted Diets   35

CHAPTER 3:   Carbohydrates—Friend or Foe?   47

PART 2 DIET

CHAPTER 4:   Your Six-Week Carb Cycling Diet Program   57

CHAPTER 5:   Your Six-Week Carb Cycling Meal Plan   75

CHAPTER 6:   Recipes for Limited-Carb Days   97

PART 3 EXERCISE

CHAPTER 7:   The Huge Benefits of Exercise   127

CHAPTER 8:   Your Six-Week Carb Cycling Exercise Program   147

CHAPTER 9:   Microcycling and Macrocycling   181

PART 4 MAINTAINING AND ADAPTATION

CHAPTER 10: The World of Sports Supplements 189

CHAPTER 11: Maintaining the Program/Common Questions
and Answers 201

CHAPTER 12: A Parting Word 209

The Carb Cycling Diet Schedule 213

Glossary 215

Resources and Suppliers 219

Bibliography 223

Index 231

About the Author 240

The CARB CYCLING DIET

Preface

Your Look Begins from Inside

It can happen around the time you celebrate your 37th or 38th birthday. Wrinkles appear on your face, you start to feel sleepy and tired at the end of the day, and you have a diminishing interest in sex or nightlife. You no longer have the strength or stamina you've been accustomed to. Worst of all, you've been on a diet and it's not working. Your body resists all efforts at weight loss, no matter how hard you try. Your goal of achieving or maintaining that youthful fit look suddenly seems impossible. Yes, you're older. But what does it mean? It means that your body has started to produce fewer anabolic hormones: Human Growth Hormone (HGH), DHEA, and testosterone. Anabolic hormones stimulate building processes, cell growth, and renewal. These hormones give us energy, vitality, lean bodies, and elastic, wrinkle-free skin. In the following chapters you will learn that as we age our body produces less and less anabolic hormones, and balance gradually shifts towards catabolism. That is why aging brings muscle loss, bone loss, wrinkled skin. Right away you may ask: How can I increase levels of anabolic hormones and prevent that decline?

To increase anabolic hormone levels, anti-aging doctors recommend hormonal replacement therapy for men and women after 40. This type of therapy requires daily supplementation with HGH,

DHEA, and sex hormones, and may suppress your body's own hormone production. Here is good news for everyone. The Carb Cycling Diet provides a cheaper and healthier alternative to this expensive therapy. It produces even better results since it stimulates the body to produce its own anabolic hormones.

In this book you will learn how to increase levels of anabolic hormones naturally, without the burden of a high price tag. Besides increasing anabolic hormones levels, the Carb Cycling Diet invokes a wide array of positive health changes; the diet can help prevent diabetes, cardiovascular deseases, and many types of cancer.

In my practice as a sports medicine nutritionist, I see many people over the age of 35 who exercise regularly and watch their diet. They try commercial diet products, personal trainers, nutritionists, and nothing happens. They wonder why they cannot achieve the lean body they seek. I also have patients who think they can look like a model simply by changing their diet or using a new diet pill. What they do not realize is that long-term calorie restriction is working against them and only makes a bad situation worse.

I always explain to these patients that their slowed metabolism is putting breaks on their efforts. As we age, merely dieting does not give us the results we want because our bodies go through hormonal changes that slow our metabolism every year. That makes it hard to achieve goals such as fat loss or muscle building. The bottom line is, we can no longer achieve the look we want without addressing this metabolic decline.

In this book, I show how using a proven, scientific approach will increase metabolism and improve overall health. As a result, you will drop fat, build muscle, increase your energy and stamina, and improve your skin and your sex drive. You will start to feel and look younger, and the best part about it is that you don't have to give up the foods you love!

A Note about the Word "Calorie"

Everyone these days seems to be obsessed with calories, but what is a calorie, anyway? Technically, a calorie is the unit of heat required to raise the temperature of 1 gram of water by 1°C. The "calories" you eat are actually kilocalories—that is, the amount of heat required to raise the temperature of 1 kilogram of water by 1°C. However, for the purpose of readability, we refer to kilocalories in this book as simply "calories."

Four Simple Concepts

The Carb Cycling Diet rests on these four simple concepts:

1. Your body's metabolism consists of two pathways: anabolism, in which you build muscle; and catabolism, in which you burn fat. You cannot do both at the same time.

2. Therefore, you need to alternate between normal-carb days (which promote anabolism) and limited-carb days (which promote catabolism). Keep in mind that when we talk about limiting carbs, we're talking primarily about refined (bad) carbs.

3. However, when you consume carbs on your normal-carb days, you also open the door to fat deposition, which usually takes place within the first few minutes of eating refined carbs.

4. In order to prevent that fat deposition, on normal-carb days, anaerobic weight lifting exercises are most effective. On limited-carb days, aerobic exercises are most effective.

Later, these concepts will be more fully examined.

We hear so much about the Atkins Diet, the South Beach Diet, and other low-carb diets, it's easy to forget that carbohydrates are actually good for you. This book employs a disciplined approach to incorporating carbs into your diet and teaches you how to use them effectively to fight fat and build muscle. It will also give you an integrated exercise plan. Diet and exercise can be used separately or in conjunction with each other, but when both are combined intelligently into one program, and work together, they create the most powerful tool you can find to fight fat.

Science

The CARB CYCLING DIET

Creating a Diet That Really Works: The Proven Power of the Carb Cycling Diet

The Carb Cycling Diet does not promise instant miracles. The truth of the matter is that the full power of the diet—and the benefits of fat loss it provides—develops gradually over a period of time. The full benefits cannot show up until your insulin secretion comes down. As you will learn later in this book, insulin is the primary hormone responsible for fat deposition. Reducing insulin secretion takes time to happen and the time varies with each person. For some it takes days and others a few weeks before the first sign of diminished insulin secretion, a diminished appetite, appears. After that happens, your protein-rich, limited-carb days will become efficient fat-loss days.

Here's what will be happening. Many years of undisciplined eating caused your pancreas to secrete large amounts of insulin, even between meals. Freely eaten snacks, bread, and sweets create a constant need for insulin secretions. How does that affect your health? Slowly but surely it begins to wear out your pancreas, predisposing you to develop type 2 diabetes. Along with undisciplined eating comes an array of cardiovascular complications in the heart and blood vessels.

As You Age, You Must Change Your Lifestyle

Why, you may ask, don't young people suffer dire consequences from eating so many carbs, including fattening refined carbs? The main reason is because young people generate high levels of protective hormones—Human Growth Hormone (HGH), thyroid, and sex hormones. Because of their high metabolism, the sugar-water glucose in their blood burns up before it gets a chance to be deposited as fat. When you are young, those surging hormones are your protective shield. When age lowers the hormone supply, the level of protection drops. That's why middle age opens the door to disease and the age-related loss of muscle and bone.

Can we reverse life's inevitable metabolic decline? No, but we can at least slow this aging tendency. The older you become the more effort you need to put in to prevent a sharp decline in anabolic hormone secretion. This can be done via increasing the amount of strength-training exercises, such as weight lifting, and diminishing the amount of aerobic exercise, such as running. A true Fountain of Youth may only exist in fairy tales, but as you read on you will see how the Carb Cycling Diet can help you stay younger longer and look your best at any age.

What Is Metabolism, Anyway?

Everyone seems to want to "boost their metabolism" these days, but do you know why or exactly what metabolism is, anyway? Metabolism is simply a set of biochemical reactions that take place inside the body. This is the area where the Carb Cycling Diet concentrates its attention. Metabolism is the sum of all biochemical processes involved in life, the process by which energy is produced. Metabolism follows two pathways: catabolism (destroying) and anabolism (building). Usually these two pathways match each other so that there is no net loss or gain. But there are conditions under which one dominates over the other. For now it is important simply to know that the body is constantly in the process of disintegrating and rejuvenating itself, destroying and rebuilding its cells and tissues. The more active this process, the faster the turnover and the younger you feel and look. This is what is meant by having "a fast metabolism." Aging and prolonged calorie restriction slows down this turnover. This is exactly what the Carb Cycling Diet is designed to prevent.

Anabolism increases synthesis of protein. Anabolism is the process by which simple food substances—glucose, fatty acids, and amino acids—are changed into living tissue: flexing biceps and fulsome lips. When you eat more calories than you burn, the balance becomes positive. That condition lets your body build proteins more efficiently, which builds muscles and connective tissue. Unfortunately, fat deposition occurs at the same time. Later in the book you will learn how to maintain your muscle while preventing fat deposition. Catabolism, meanwhile, breaks down tissues and leads to fat loss.

The action of metabolism is controlled by hormones. They are metabolism's traffic cops. The balance between catabolism and anabolism is controlled by anabolic hormones (Human Growth Hormone, testosterone) on one side and catabolic hormones (cortisol, glucagon) on the other side.

If your body produces higher levels of anabolic hormones, that translates into a higher rate of anabolic metabolism—more protein is produced. If it produces small amounts of anabolic hormones, it means less protein is produced and, as a result, your body has a

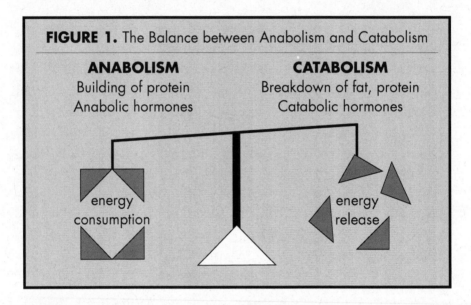

FIGURE 1. The Balance between Anabolism and Catabolism

ANABOLISM
Building of protein
Anabolic hormones

CATABOLISM
Breakdown of fat, protein
Catabolic hormones

energy consumption

energy release

slower rate of tissue repair. The sagging, wrinkled skin, small muscles, and fragile bones of old age are the result.

Let's look at how anabolism and catabolism work together. Most of the time, when the calories you consume equal your Daily Calorie Needs, they balance each other out so there is no gain or loss of living tissue. But there are situations when one dominates over the other. In Negative Calorie Balance, catabolism dominates and leads to fat and protein loss. In Positive Calorie Balance, anabolism dominates and leads to fat and protein gain.

Controlling this balance by alternating anabolism with catabolism is the key to the Carb Cycling Diet.

Consider this simple equation.

Calories You Eat – Calories You Burn = Calorie Balance

When you consume fewer calories than you use, the balance becomes negative and you are in a catabolic state, in which catabolism dominates over anabolism. Catabolism leads to weight loss, which is made up of fat loss, muscle loss, water loss, and bone loss. When you eat the same amount of calories that you burn, the balance becomes zero. Anabolism and catabolism balance out each other and you can not lose weight.

THE FOUR ELEMENTS OF METABOLISM

To understand metabolism we should get to know its four elements: 1) basal metabolic rate, 2) exercise and other physical activity, 3) digestion of food, and 4) adaptive heat generation. Let's look at each more closely.

Basal metabolic rate (BMR): This is the number of calories the body burns at rest. This amounts to about 65 to 70 percent of total metabolism. As a rough gauge, some nutritionists say that basal metabolic rate burns about ten calories for each pound of body weight. So a 135 pound person would burn 1,350 calories a day just by staying all day in bed.

Exercise and other physical activity: This is the amount of calories burned during all activity in a 24-hour period. Exercise accounts for 15 to 25 percent of total metabolism. Your goal should be 25 percent.

Digestion of food: This is the amount of calories burned during the digestion and absorption of food. It accounts for 5 to 10 percent of total metabolism.

Adaptive heat generation: These are the calories used to produce body heat and keep body temperature regulated. It accounts for about 7 percent of total metabolism.

Here is how these elements work together:

Basal metabolic rate (65 to 70 percent)
+ Physical activity (15 to 25 percent)
+ Food digestion (5 to 10 percent)
+ Temperature control (7 percent)

= Total metabolism (100 percent)

Your total metabolism equals your Daily Calorie Needs. If you consume calories equal to your Daily Calorie Needs, the balance would be zero and no fat loss or fat gain would occur.

The Role of Hormones

Biochemists understand the process of glucose metabolism, but they aren't clear on why some people can eat large amounts of sugar and refined carbohydrates and not gain weight while some people are not so lucky. Why, for instance, can a 16-year-old eat pizza, ice cream, and cookies, and gulp 32-ounce cola drinks—consuming more than 3,000 calories a day—and still maintain five-percent body fat? The same number of calories consumed later in life would lead to swift obesity. The answer lies in the mysterious world of hormones, which work as traffic policemen to tell your body what to do and when to accelerate the speed of metabolic reactions.

Here are the main hormones involved in metabolism. Human Growth Hormone (HGH) is a primary anabolic hormone, produced by a small gland inside the brain. This hormone and its metabolites stimulate all cells to grow and divide. As we age, HGH levels decline. Testosterone is another major anabolic hormone that is responsible for male attributes such as a lean, muscular body. Some testosterone is found in women's bodies also. In women, it plays an important role in evoking a sexual desire. Estrogen, a female hormone, can be found in men's bodies as well. (Incidentally, estrogen levels in men increase, as a result of the increasing conversion of testosterone into estrogen as they age, accompanied by a decline in testosterone.) Blood concentration and a balance of sex hormones have been identified as playing an important role in the regulation of fat distribution. The problematic area fat cells have sex hormone receptors that react on testosterone and estrogen changes by storing or releasing fat.

HGH, testosterone, and insulin (which we'll discuss in more detail later) work primarily on the anabolic, or "growth," portion of your body's metabolism, so they are known as anabolic hormones.

The thyroid hormone is a multifunctional hormone (it affects both anabolic and catabolic actions) that is involved in many metabolic reactions. It regulates body temperature, stimulates the nervous system, and enhances protein, carbohydrate, and fat utilization. Its anabolic actions are more evident during childhood and teenage development.

Cortisol is a catabolic hormone produced by the adrenal glands. The level of this hormone is increased during stressful situations; for example, during heavy exercise, emotional stress, or when blood glucose concentration drops. It helps to stabilize blood glucose levels by utilizing proteins for energy. Cortisol is responsible for muscle loss.

Glucagon is another catabolic hormone that is produced by the pancreas in response to low blood glucose concentration. It raises the glucose level by mobilizing glucose from glycogen. It also speeds up the conversion of amino acids into glucose, thus leading to the breakdown of protein.

THYROID HORMONES AND THE METABOLIC RATE

The thyroid gland regulates the metabolic rate. How does this work? A thyroid hormone, thyroxine, is created by combining the amino acid tyrosine with iodine. Thyroxine increases the number and activity of mitochondria in cells. Mitochondria is the energy-producing unit of the cell.

The thyroid hormones accelerate the rate of both anabolism and catabolism. Studies of obese women have shown that a certain percentage of women are suffering from an inactive thyroid gland. When their thyroid hormone levels were restored to normal these women showed a significant fat loss. Mary, a 38-year-old woman who was 5'6",185 pounds, complained of tiredness, low energy, depression, feeling cold all the time, and an irregular menstrual cycle. She said that she watched her diet by staying away from sweets. She asked me if an exercise program could help her to regain the lost vitality. The blood test showed subnormal thyroid hormones levels. I advised her to supplement with kelp, L-tyrosine, Coenzyme Q-10, and include some carbohydrates in her diet to increase thyroid gland activity. She responded within a week with increased energy and mood. The repeated blood test showed normal levels of thyroid hormones.

Women should check their thyroid hormone level before initiating a fat-loss program. Thyroid hormone supplementation should be done only under a doctor's supervision since it carries a potential for overdosing. There is a safe way of stimulating thyroid gland function by supplementation with L-tyrosine and kelp, which we'll cover in Chapter 10.

Insulin and Glucose Uptake

After you eat, the glucose level in your blood rises, which triggers the pancreas to secrete insulin. Insulin opens glucose transport channels located on a cell's membranes. This is called insulin-stimulated glucose uptake and it's an important concept to those involved in dieting. The insulin causes a thirty-fold increase in the rate of glucose uptake by the body cells.

Insulin is an anabolic hormone. It enables nutrients to enter cells and provide building blocks necessary for protein synthesis. It is also one of the most important hormones in the weight-loss equation. When the insulin level is high, glucose enters fat cells (adipose tissue) and is deposited there as triglycerides (TG). In contrast, when the insulin level is low, triglycerides break down to fatty acids that exit fat cells and are used as an energy source.

Glucose is a simple sugar and the product of the digestion of carbohydrates. Glucose is a single sugar molecule (monosaccharide) related to table sugar (sucrose). Your body has a regulatory mechanism to keep its blood glucose concentration constant. When the blood glucose concentration rises, the pancreas secretes a hormone called insulin that decreases the sugar concentration by pushing the glucose into body cells.

What would happen if blood glucose were not regulated? The blood concentration might reach such high levels at which the osmotic ingredient in glucose would attract water to the blood vessels, leaving cell tissues dehydrated. That action would lead to death. On the other hand, a feeble level of blood glucose is not advisable because glucose must be present in blood to support the healthy functioning of red blood cells, nerve cells, and many organs.

THE AMAZING GLYCOGEN MOLECULE

An important thing to know about glycogen is that it's formed by animals—not plants—and it serves as a repository of glucose. It could be argued that glucose (sugar water) is to glycogen what money is to a bank. The liver and muscle tissues are collection points and holding places for glycogen. It can be looked at this way. Glucose is deposited in three places: the Liver Bank, the Muscle Bank, and the Fat Cells Bank. The glucose can be deposited as fat in fat cells and as glycogen in muscles and liver. At this point, it is important to know that the liver and muscles convert sugar-water glucose into glycogen for storage and later use as an energy reserve. This concept is crucial to the Carb Cycling Diet.

The liver contains sufficient reserves of glycogen for an overnight fast. If you do not eat carbohydrates for more than 12 hours, the glycogen reserves in your liver have been depleted. Some carbohydrates eaten for breakfast will be transformed into liver glycogen to restore its reserves that were used during night fast. This is one of the reasons why we recommend consuming refined carbs in the morning, especially for those who do not exercise.

Muscle glycogen provides instant, easily accessible energy to muscles. As molecules go, the glycogen molecule is extremely large. (Technically, it is a complex, branched-chain polysaccharide.) This has an important cosmetic effect for people with a large glycogen bankroll. The accumulation of big glycogen molecules in the muscles has a plumping effect that makes the muscles look larger. Part of those bulging biceps in body builder Arnold Schwarzenegger is an ample supply of muscle glycogen. Follow the Carb Cycling Diet and you can take advantage of the same scientific principle he used to build those bulging muscles.

Glycogen also enables a muscle to generate a rapid release of energy. That capability is particularly important when the oxygen in the blood is insufficient to supply the muscle's instant demand for energy. This happens during periods of forceful muscle contraction—when exercise is performed at high intensity. If muscles suddenly need energy, such as during a 200-meter Olympic sprint, most of that energy called upon will be delivered from the anaerobic breakdown of muscle glycogen. It's a runaround solution to a waning oxygen supply.

How to Lose Fat and Build Protein

Rule 1: Losing Fat = Catabolism

You cannot lose fat unless you are in a Negative Calorie Balance and catabolism is dominant.

Rule 2: Building Protein = Anabolism

You cannot build extra protein (muscle and connective tissues) unless you are in a Positive Calorie Balance and anabolism is dominant.

Rule 3: Fat and Muscle

Since anabolism and catabolism cannot be dominant simultaneously we cannot lose fat and build muscle on the same day.

While you cannot lose fat and build protein on the same day, you can achieve both goals by alternating the days in which you lose fat with the days in which you effectively build protein. You must alternate periods of catabolism, or Negative Calorie Balance when you lose fat, with periods of anabolism, or Positive Calorie Balance when your body builds proteins and effectively rejuvenates its tissues. This alternating process is the very core of the Carb Cycling Diet.

HOW TO LOSE FAT IN A HEALTHY WAY

Using diet pills and skin patches to suppress appetite is a popular way to lose fat, but in the long run pills and patches don't work. As soon as people stop taking them, their appetite returns, followed by the return of fat. So what is the solution? If you want to lose fat in a healthy way, you should alternate between catabolism and anabolism.

Catabolism allows you to lose weight by reducing your caloric intake below your Daily Calorie Needs. To lose fat in a healthy way, you need to periodically make anabolism dominate over catabolism. Even short periods of anabolic dominance can create a condition in which the body puts off muscle and bone destruction, effectively repairs micro and macrotraumas, and restores normal levels of vital hormones.

HOW TO BUILD PROTEIN IN A HEALTHY WAY

How do you make anabolism dominate over catabolism? Periodically boost exercise intensity together with eating enough calories to force your body to release anabolic hormones. The special MAX effort exercise, described later in Chapter 8, can help you to increase your level of anabolic hormones. If you are unable to perform the MAX effort exercise for any reason, simply do any type of exercise at a higher intensity than normal. Follow this basic rule: When increasing intensity, decrease exercise time and vice versa.

Anabolism synthesizes hormones and other complex substances and gives your body a youth-preserving boost. During anabolism, your body can repair broken chains of proteins more effectively. It can better renew proteins, such as those in the skin and cartilage. Without these extra calories and a hormonal boost, the rate of repair of elastin and collagen slows down every year. If we don't take measures to counteract slow metabolism, we begin to look old and fat. The Carb Cycling Diet allows you to achieve a healthy balance between trimming off fat and keeping your body looking and feeling young longer.

Metabolism and Aging

As we age, we lose bone and muscle mass and accumulate fat. In other words, we become flabby and obese. If we try to counteract this fat gain by following a traditional diet that simply reduces calorie intake, it makes a bad situation worse. Traditional dieting slows down metabolism, which is already impaired by aging. Inadequate nutrition, reduced food intake, and a sedentary lifestyle accelerate muscle loss, bone loss, wrinkle formation, and a decrease in the production of the vital anabolic hormones—HGH, testosterone, and DHEA. Calorie restriction through dieting slows many important rejuvenation processes in our bodies that take place every day and accelerates development of degenerative conditions of aging.

As you age, catabolism comes to dominate over anabolism. Therefore, you need to speed up your metabolism as you age so you can prevent fat accumulation and prolong your vitality—not to slow it as the fad diets mistakenly do.

The CARB CYCLING DIET

The Problem with Calorie Restricted Diets

A new millennium has arrived and everyone thinks they know how to lose fat. After all, this generation is the most sophisticated and best educated in the history of the world. And there are hundreds of diets and diet products on the market. Yet, more than half of all Americans are overweight—many are obese. Why? Something is drastically wrong.

Any food restriction, whether it comes from protein, carbohydrates, or fat, will lead to fat loss in the beginning. This initial fat loss is always the easiest and fastest. That is why so many diets claim that you can lose 20 pounds with minimum effort. Many people do. But the initial fat loss stops short before one is able to lose "problem area" fat unless the dieter undertakes severe restrictions. What is wrong with going deeper in food restriction? Gradually, these people lose muscle and bone mass and develop nutritional deficiencies that affect all aspects of their life—energy level, sex drive, immune system response, skin elasticity, joint health, bone density, and more.

Deprivation Diets Simply Don't Work

Ask a group of athletes if they can perform their best while they are being denied carbohydrates. They'll laugh at you. Have you ever heard of an athlete who follows the Atkins or other low-carb diet? When it comes to physical activities, carbohydrates are essential energy sources.

This is why the "eat less, exercise more" concept, if taken blindly, can actually work against you, especially as you age. First of all, your body needs more nutrients and more calories when you start an exercise program to effectively repair any micro-traumas, especially in joints and muscles. Prolonged calories or food restriction leads to nutritional deficiencies. Secondly, studies show that people lose protein (muscles) even while exercising on calorie-restricted diets. Thirdly, a high volume of exercise on calorie-restricted diets suppresses the release of anabolic hormones, slows down your metabolism, and leads to overtraining. Overtraining is a metabolic condition resulted from excessive exercise without adequate periods of rest. Rest days are important component of the Carb Cycling Diet exercise program. If at any time you feel tired or sleepy, lose interest in exercise, or perform worse, you are probably on the edge of overtraining; take a few days of rest. Sometimes a week or two are necessary.

Here's an example of one of my patients, Steve, a 40-year-old man, 5'10" tall, and 172 pounds. He exercised regularly five days a week by running for 20 to 40 minutes. He also alternated lifting weights with playing tennis or bicycling. He followed a restricted calorie low-carb Atkins diet model. He complained that by 9 PM he was exhausted. Going to bed early did not make him feel more rested. He also had lost interest in sex and asked me to prescribe Cialis because he and his wife wanted a second child. He also wanted to improve his running performance.

I took his blood for analysis. The results showed that his levels of HGH and testosterone were low. The physical examinations revealed that he had 19 percent body fat. He said that when he started running he lost 16 pounds but his muscles seemed to shrink. All of these were signs to me that his body was deeply in a catabolic state and his metabolism had slowed down significantly. Right away he asked me: "Why is my metabolism running slow if I exercise regularly and eat a healthy diet?" It took me some time to explain to him that long-term calorie restriction plus exercise forced his body into self-destroying catabolic mode. His body was not producing enough testosterone and other building hormones and many of his vital functions were beginning to suffer. Steve was not aware of two important facts: Too much aerobic exercise conditions the cardiovascular system but, if performed without adequate protection from the damaging effects of free radicals, contributes to aging. If accompanied with prolonged calorie restriction, it also leads to suppression of anabolic hormone production.

What were my recommendations? Stop the Atkins diet. Increase calorie and carbohydrate intake, and take two weeks off from exercising. After that I said he should engage in weight lifting and anabolic hormone-releasing exercises to boost his testosterone (among other anabolic hormones). As we age we tend to secrete fewer and fewer anabolic hormones. This process is gradual and happens unnoticeably until the time when we finally realize that something is not as used to be. After only two months, Steve sent me a note thanking me for bringing his life back on track. His energy level and metabolism skyrocketed and his wife got pregnant (without any Cialis).

As Steve's example shows, this is the looming problem for those on a calorie-restricted diet for a prolonged period of time. Unknowingly, they suffer from undernutrition (a form of malnutrition), lowered levels of anabolic hormones, and a weakening of the immune system—the body's first line of defense against cancer and infections. The average American is not consuming anywhere near the amount of fruit and vegetables recommended by the American Dietary Association, even those who are not on a calorie-restricted diet. What happens when the amount of food he or she eats is artificially restricted? The body does not receive adequate amounts of active nutrients, vitamins, minerals, bioflavonoids, etc. By the way, those who exercise need even more nutrients that those who are not.

Some may say a daily multivitamin pill will cover up for nutritional gaps. It does not. The best multivitamin and mineral formula has only a small percentage of the wide spectrum of nutrients found in natural foods. The importance of consuming an adequate amount and variety of food is obvious to any nutritionist or medical doctor.

Here are just a few of the negative physiological consequences that result from long-term calorie deprivation.

Slow metabolism (diminished BMR): The opposite of the desired goal. The body adjusts to a lower calorie intake by diminishing BMR.

Lack of libido: Fewer anabolic hormones are produced. The body produces less HGH, tesosterone, DHEA, thyroid hormones when are not enough calories available.

Depression: The low levels of testosterone has been shown to be link to depression in men.

Wrinkles: Connective tissue proteins have broken down and do not repair effectively. Under catabolic dominance, the body breaks down more proteins than it builds, including those in the skin.

Joint pain: The breakdown of cartilage, resulting from micro-traumas from exercise.

Hair loss: A result of connective tissue protein breakdown. Hair follicles lose connective tissue support.

Muscle loss: Studies show that 25 percent of weight loss is muscle tissue.

Accelerated osteoporosis: Bone loss is a result of a loss of calcium. Studies show that people on low-carb diets lose as much as 130 milligrams of calcium a day. Calcium is essential to the proper functioning of every cell in your body. The heartbeat, muscle contractions, the hormone system, the functioning of your brain, your eyes and ears—all depend on calcium. It also plays a critical role in blood clotting and cell division, and of course, in keeping your bones and teeth strong.

Nothing can cure osteoporosis. The key is prevention, which includes adequate calcium intake early in life and plenty of exercise throughout life. The best sources of calcium are milk, cheese, dairy products, dark green leafy vegetables, beans, and peas. Put these foods on your approved list. Calcium supplements are also helpful, but shouldn't replace calcium intake from food sources. A repetitive and regular load on bones (such as weight lifting and jumping) also makes the bones stronger.

The Benefits of the Carb Cycling Diet

So what are the benefits of the Carb Cycling Diet?

1. The diet reduces refined carbohydrate consumption. That alone gives your pancreas the luxury of a well-needed rest.
2. It prevents a rapid slowdown in metabolism.
3. It prevents loss of protein, ensuring that you will not be debilitated by atrophied muscles and osteoarthritis when you reach your retirement years.
4. It prevents fat deposition by depleting glycogen levels.
5. Through exercise, the Carb Cycling Diet boosts the level of anabolic hormones (HGH, growth factors, and testosterone).
6. It slows down aging and prevents age-related diseases.

REDUCING REFINED CARBS

Many people continue to ask me why I concentrate on refined carbohydrates. Why not on fat? The answer is pretty simple. Refined carbohydrates trigger an insulin secretion, which plays an important role in building fat deposits and controlling blood sugar that influences the onset of hunger. At first, eating refined carbohydrates makes you feel full and satisfied. Soon after that, a new wave of hunger strikes. While calorie restriction remains the most important factor in fat loss, carbohydrate restriction makes it easier to eat less food. That's because a lower level of insulin diminishes hunger. Another reason for restricting refined carb intake? Restricting refined carbs does not deprive your body of any essential nutrients.

Refined carbohydrates are the basis for many of our pleasure foods. We tend to eat pleasure foods in such large quantities that the number of calories we consume exceeds the amount we burn for energy. Most of our pleasure foods—white bread, cookies, cakes and ice cream—are loaded with refined carbohydrates, which quickly break down into glucose, a blood sugar and a very powerful energy source. Like nuclear fuel, refined carbohydrates, if managed properly, provide useful energy. Yet, if either is left uncontrolled, they can lead to disaster.

Here's a thing or two you should know about carbs. Highly refined carbs like pasta, sugar, bread and cake, digest almost instantly. When they hit the bloodstream, they trigger the pancreas gland to squirt a shot of insulin into the bloodstream. The purpose of the insulin is to carry that cake-turned-sugar-water to the body's cells to be used as energy or to be stored as fat.

When you consume refined carbohydrates, you touch off a storm reaction in your body. The storm sends waves of insulin coursing through the bloodstream. It takes time before the insulin stabilizes and returns to its original level. During that wild ride, many things happen: nutrients move through cell membranes, the blood glucose level drops, producing a craving for more sweets. While refined carbohydrates give us a sense of well-being, in the long run they damage the internal organs. For example, too much glucose and insulin can result in fatty deposits on the walls of the blood vessels and that can eventually clog them and lead to hypertension, stroke, or a heart attack (myocardial infarction). We may not suffer a heart attack within minutes of eating a piece of birthday cake, but years of bingeing on refined carbohydrates can accumulate and eventually do a lot of damage.

Is sugar a poison? Many medical and nutritional authorities label sugar as a silent killer. Over a lifetime, sugar helps kill people. Eating refined carbs every day puts a stress on the pancreas that eventually can lead to its failure.

What about a low-fat diet? It works because it dramatically restricts calories. A low-fat diet operates on the principle that fat is bad for you and carbohydrates are good for you. Yet fat is essential to good health. And on a low-fat diet, people often overeat carbohydrates, which have a negative impact on human health.

PREVENTING A SLOWDOWN IN YOUR METABOLISM

I'm sure you've heard that if your calorie intake exceeds your calorie expenditure, the unused calories will turn to fat. In other words, if you deduct the number of calories you burn from the number of calories you eat, you have the number of calories that will turn to fat. That's not quite right. That formula fails to take into account two important calorie storage places—the muscle and liver glycogen depots—that can absorb calories. The Carb Cycling Diet will teach you how to use these two calorie storage places for your personal benefit. And that makes all the difference between the Carb Cycling Diet and the others.

Many of my patients complain that they eat 500 fewer calories than their daily needs and lose no weight. The common practice among nutritionists is to advise the dieter to lower calorie intake by 500 calories and expect to see one pound of fat loss each week. (A pound of fat contains 3,500 calories.) It just doesn't work for long. The body quickly adapts by lowering its basal metabolic rate (BMR) so the calorie-deficit disappears. The BMR, the number of calories necessary to maintain your body's basic functions at rest, is the number of calories your body need if you stay in bed 24 hours.

As you can see, the simple mathematical calculation of input and output that we have been taught to rely on is not accurate. Our body has complex regulatory and adaptation mechanisms. The secret of the Carb Cycling Diet is to work with these mechanisms—and not against them. Nutrition is not a precise science based on mathematics, even though many nutrition advisers would have you think so. There are mechanisms that usually are not accounted for by the conventional dieting approach, the body's adaptation and self-regulation. This diet and exercise program will concentrate on these mechanisms.

The Carb Cycling Diet aims at preventing the adaptation changes that occur when someone's behavior becomes repetitious. For example, when someone consumes a calorie-restricted diet day after day for months on end, the body adjusts to this calorie deficit by lowering its expectations. It slows metabolism. When someone performs the same exercise day after day, the body adjusts and starts hoarding calories. Knowing this allows you to take preventive actions.

PREVENTING LOSS OF PROTEIN

All fad diets have a similar idea: reduce the number of calories the dieter consumes. What effect does that have down the road? It may not be noticeable until you spend a year on the diet. There are ample studies to show that 25 percent of dietary weight loss comes from the loss of muscle tissues. In short, losing fat is accompanied by losing muscle.

Do we lose protein selectively from the muscles? The answer is a definite no. Besides muscle protein, there is a loss of connective tissue protein—those called elastin and collagen. The connective-tissue proteins are what make your skin firm and elastic. They are nature's own Botox. The loss of these proteins makes your skin sag and creates wrinkles. The connective tissue proteins are also part of joint cartilage and ligaments. The loss of it can lead to joint pains and osteoarthrosis, a degenerative condition of the joints.

Take a look at anyone over the age of 35 who has been on a calorie-restricted diet for a year or more. Even though they've lost weight, the skin on their face became wrinkled and is no more elastic as used to be. Is it simply aging or it is something they are doing wrong? I am sure they could look and feel much better if they take a different approach to diet and exercise. You can look and feel better than your age by following simple steps: periodically boost your calorie intake and exercise to stimulate anabolic hormone secretion. The Carb Cycling Diet will give you guidelines on how to do it.

PREVENTING FAT DEPOSITION

The Carb Cycling Diet employs two body mechanisms to prevent fat deposition from taking place:
1. It brings down the level of glycogen, a condition which allows you to eat carbohydrates.
2. It keeps insulin levels stable on limited-carb days, which prevents new fat deposition.

This strategy is preventive. It is harder to get rid of your love handles than it is to prevent the fat from landing there in the first place. Use carbohydrate cycling to keep your insulin level stable most days of the week. In that way no fat deposition can take place.

On limited-carb days you need to consume increased amounts of protein. You can also get essential amino acids by taking supplements. Increased amino acids intake prevents muscle loss. You may wish to augment your diet with branched-chain amino acids, called BCAA. They are available in capsule form from health food stores. Take two to four capsules of BCAA between each meal and at nighttime, or whenever you feel hungry. The capsule form is convenient to carry when you're on the go.

The better commercial whey protein also contains BCAA, so you needn't take both on the same day. The branched-chain amino acids ward off hunger while providing essential amino acids. This way your body gets essential amino acids without increased fat intake of meat. It is also suitable for vegetarians. If you're at work or at home, have a whey protein shake or mix it with your favorite nonfat yogurt. If you're away, take a few BCAA capsules.

Managing your food intake is an ongoing process. Many people tell themselves "I'll eat a cookie now and later in the day I'll burn it off at the gym." That's not a great tactic. You might not get to the gym. More importantly, fat is deposited as soon as you eat refined carbs, not at the end of the day. By the time you get to the gym, it's too late. You've got another layer on your love handles. Now you must exercise twice as hard to force the body to shed those fat reserves.

There is a way to keep that cookie from turning into fat. Simply exercise before eating the cookie. Under these circumstances, the glucose derived from the cookie—if not used right away for energy—will enter muscle tissue or liver cells and be deposited there as glycogen instead of turning into fat.

The liver glycogen serves as a major reserve for keeping the blood glucose level constant. In between meals, when there is no incoming glucose from food, the liver glycogen keeps blood glucose from falling dangerously low. As we've discussed, the amount in the liver is just enough to get you through a 12-hour fast. When reserves of glycogen are depleted, the body starts to break down protein. Some amino acids can be converted into glucose. This is how we lose valuable muscle tissue. To prevent protein breakdown, I recommend eating unrefined carbohydrates in small equal portions throughout the day so blood glucose never drops too low and body will not be forced to convert amino acids into glucose. Eating small portions of Healthy Breakfast (a recipe for which appears in Chapter 6) throughout the day serves this purpose.

The amount of glycogen stored in muscles can vary. The larger the muscles, the more they can store. Muscle glycogen serves as a primary source of energy for as much as 20 minutes of intense exercise. Then muscle glycogen is depleted. The body will try to restore glycogen as soon as it has a chance. That means any carbohydrate you eat after exercise will be deposited as glycogen and not as fat. That's good news. The Carb Cycling Diet recommends consuming refined carbs within 2 hours after the exercise. During this time window you can have a few meals with refined carbohydrates.

Boosting Anabolic Hormones through Exercise

A high intensity exercise leads to release of anabolic hormones. If performed regularly it stimulates internal glands to keep producing increased amounts of these vital hormones. In the long run, it is very advantageous since it protects your health, has anti-aging effects, and improves your level of fitness.

From this perspective, a short but intensive exercise session is superior to a long and non-intensive exercise session. It does not matter what type of exercise (cardiovascular, strength-training, etc.), only that it is of high intensity. But be aware that a high intensity should be used sparingly. Too much of it can lead to overtraining, when the body slows the production of anabolic hormones. Make sure that your program has no more than one or two high intensity days a week with days of rest in between.

SLOWING DOWN AGING

Here are three key factors on how the Carb Cycling Diet slows down aging:

1. It creates a Positive Calorie Balance that is a necessary condition to stimulate anabolism. As you learned earlier in the book, in order to stay young you need to accelerate metabolism, particularly anabolism. The body would not produce large amounts of anabolic hormones if it does not have enough calories. On the other hand, just eating large quantities of calories, without intensive exercise, would not increase your anabolic hormone levels. That is why the next factor is important.

2. It recommends intensive weight lifting, which builds muscles and boosts anabolic hormone secretion. You will learn later in this book how to exercise in order to increase an anabolic hormone secretion.

3. It utilizes supplements as necessary, which increase energy and endurance and fight free radicals. During exercise, free radicals are produced in increased amounts. Many studies have showed that free radicals, highly active molecules that are usually the product of oxygen metabolism, can cause premature aging and even cancer.

These three factors combat the negative physiological changes that accompany human aging. You might say they provide a key to the Fountain of Youth.

The CARB CYCLING DIET

3

Carbohydrates—
Friend or Foe?

Carbohydrates make food sweet and satisfying, which is why we can eat them and easily surpass our daily calorie limit. In addition, refined carbs possess the highest insulin-invoking potential of any food. As you have read, insulin is the blackest villain in making fat deposits.

To humans, carbohydrates mean energy. Carbs become important when you need energy to perform physical activities. There are two kinds of carbohydrates: refined carbohydrates, which are generally bad for you, and unrefined carbohydrates, which are generally good for you. The type of carbohydrate you eat determines how quickly this energy becomes available and how long it will last. Refined carbohydrates generally represent our pleasure foods—cake and glazed doughnuts—and they deliver a quick burst of glucose to your blood. It is a quick fix: This happens within a few minutes, but the boost does not last long.

Unrefined carbohydrates are whole grains that are cracked or cut, not milled, so they retain their fiber. Oatmeal, pearl barley, and brown rice are common examples of whole grains. They digest slower and take longer to deliver energy, but the slow energy release can last several hours. The fiber slows digestion so the glucose is absorbed slowly. Therefore less insulin is secreted than that produced by the swift digestion of refined carbohydrates. This type of carbohydrates is an ideal energy source for prolonged physical activity.

Refined carbohydrates are the starches left when whole grains are highly refined through milling. Until modern milling was introduced in the 1880s, cut grains were the sole source of cereals in our diet. Until the end of the 19th century, our ancestors did not have the constantly elevated levels of insulin in their blood. Neither did they suffer from arterial plaque, heart attack, stroke, and diabetes, which are so prevalent today.

Why are so many people addicted to refined carbohydrates? For one thing, carbs are an excellent source of instant energy. In the middle of the day when the concentration of our blood glucose drops, we need an energy boost, so we go for caffeine and a soft ice cream cone. Within minutes, this carb boost gives us a sense of well-being and comfort. But it also leads to a form of physical and psychological addiction. For just one day, try going without refined carbohydrates and you will experience an irresistible craving for a carb fix. Does the body crave them for nutritional value? No, refined carbohydrates do not supply essential nutrients. We crave refined carbohydrates for the pleasant feeling they evoke, nothing more.

Many of us think that the deposition of fat takes place at the end of the day, after we go to sleep. That supposedly is the time when the body calculates the net in-and-out of calories, and puts the extra calories to one side. But the body doesn't do its math the same way our brain does. In fact, it does not calculate at all. The body senses the amount of energy molecules, called ATP, that are produced. If the amount of ATP is low, the body calls for food intake. How the body regulates its energy intake and energy expenditure is complex and not completely understood yet. This much is known, however. Research shows that most fat deposition happens in the first five minutes after eating refined carbohydrates. Yes, five minutes. That means fat deposition takes place at the point when the insulin level in your blood spikes. If there is too much glucose in the blood, insulin will force the glucose into body cells, including fat cells. The process is an ongoing balancing of energy that continues all day long. Fat deposition happens at breakfast, lunch, dinner, and snack time or any time when the glucose level is too high and your glycogen depots are full.

The body does not perform calculations at the end of the day. Rather, the energy balancing process is ongoing throughout the day. The calorie value of food serves as a guide for us to judge the energy potential the food possesses. Consume too much energy and you might run into trouble. Also keep in the mind the time factor. Bingeing on a thousand calories of ice cream in ten minutes will have a far worse impact than spreading consumption spoonful by spoonful throughout the day. The insulin spike in the first scenario will lead to instant fat deposition. If you eat the ice cream in small portions, the calories will be used for energy and not end up on your rear end as fat. That is why it is important to eat small portions throughout the day, rather than three big meals.

The source of calories can also make a difference. If you eat a 260-calorie steak and a 260-calorie candy bar, the number of calories is the same, but the results in terms of fat storage could be different. The candy bar is more fattening because its glucose touches off that stormy insulin spike. Because of that difference, a concept called the glycemic index of food was implemented.

The Glycemic Index

Not all carbs are alike. Some foods can have a relatively low amount of carbohydrates, but a high glycemic index. In that case, they make a poor choice for food. That's because even small amounts of high glycemic index carbs touch off that stormy insulin secretion.

Using the glycemic index (GI) of carbohydrates empowers you to choose between the more fattening and less fattening carbs. Refined carbs digest faster and touch off a higher insulin spike. The more refined, the higher the spike and the higher the GI index. The body digests unrefined carbs more slowly. As a result the blood absorbs the glucose more gradually and insulin level rises slowly. The insulin level might not reach a threshold value because the blood glucose is burned for energy and consequently fat deposition might not occur. That kind of carbohydrate is said to have a low glycemic index.

Establishing glycemic index levels was simple. A sample group of a dozen or so healthy adults were tested for blood sugar level, which was recorded. The volunteers were then fed a sample serving of food—boiled rice, baked potato, jelly doughnut—and after a thirty minute wait for the blood sugar level to rise, they were tested again. The increases (spikes) in the blood sugar level were averaged and that figure became the GI for that food. For example, here are some carbohydrate foods and their GIs:

> white rice—92
> baked potato—85
> French fries—75
> macaroni and cheese—64

Generally, you should choose carbs with GIs below 60. Examples include whole-wheat pasta, beans, lentils, peas, corn, carrots, nuts, and grapefruit. Be aware that GI does not take into account the amount of food eaten. For example, eating a large quantity of French fries can have a far bigger impact on insulin secretion than a moderate amount of white rice.

For a few days each week, keep your insulin level low by choosing low GI food. The goal of using the glycemic index is to bring your insulin level down to where it won't make you hungry, and won't force you to binge. That's why it is important to pay close attention to the GI in the beginning of the program, when your insulin level is still high. Later, when the insulin level comes down, focus more attention on the amount of calories consumed each day. As we've said, try to choose foods with a GI lower than 60. You need not avoid all carbohydrates. Unprocessed carbohydrates are good sources of fiber and energy.

On some occasions our body does need refined carbohydrates because refined carbs provide an instant energy source, especially for your muscles, and invoke the highest insulin secretion, which allows nutrients to quickly enter the cells.

Carbohydrates + Fat = Bad Deal

Because of the surge of insulin, refined carbohydrates and fat are a bad food combination. The Carb Cycling Diet equips you with the knowledge that you can eat well for the rest of your life, no matter what. Keep these guidelines in your mind:

Refined carbohydrates + fat = bad choice
Unprocessed carbohydrates + fat = okay

As we age, our body's sensitivity to insulin changes. Each cell in our body carries insulin receptors. When someone eats too many refined carbs and produces a continually high level of insulin, these receptors stop reacting; they become unresponsive. Suddenly, the body becomes insulin resistant.

What can we do about this unhealthy development? We need to bring down our insulin secretion. Taking a break from the carb overload we experience every day would be a first healthy step to undertake. The first six weeks on the Carb Cycling Diet are specifically focused on lowering insulin secretion. Regular exercise will help too. The studies show that those who exercise regularly improve insulin sensitivity. Muscles consume large quantity of glucose from the blood thus diminishing blood glucose concentration.

The Carb Cycling Diet is based on an on-off consumption of carbohydrates, especially refined carbohydrates. When coupled with regular exercise, it helps to achieve and keep a desired body shape. While this dietary approach can be used without an exercise program, by far the best results occur when the user combines the two. Even if you cannot find time for exercise, you still can apply the carbohydrate cycling strategy to keep your body fit and healthy.

Diet

The CARB CYCLING DIET

4

Your Six-Week Carb Cycling Diet Program

Now that you have a basic understanding of what anabolism and catabolism are and how your metabolism works, along with the powerful role of hormones and the dramatic impact of refined carbs, let's put it all together into a diet plan that will help you lose fat and build a lean body.

The Carb Cycling Diet is so flexible that you can adjust it to literally any lifestyle. The main advantage is that it gives you the luxury of eating pleasurable food in a controlled and managed way. You eat refined carbs—the target food—on some days and avoid them on others. When to eat it is extremely important.

As you've also learned, the Carb Cycling Diet will protect you from the debilitating conditions of aging such as muscle loss, osteoporosis, as well as thickened artery walls, diabetes, breast and colon cancer, stroke, and heart attack. If you complement this diet with an exercise program, the benefits will be even greater.

Carb Cycling Regimens

It's a proven fact that restricting carbohydrates is an effective way to wage war against fat, but following such an extreme low-carb diet, such as Atkins, can become difficult because you must avoid all those tempting refined-carb foods for the rest of your life. Most people lose fat initially but fail to maintain the diet long enough and thus gain back the fat.

On the Carb Cycling Diet, alternating between catabolism (fat breakdown) and anabolism (tissue building), is not only healthier, but gives you more flexibility and is easier to maintain long term. As soon as you became accustomed to this alternate cycling pattern, you can adjust your level of carbohydrate consumption to suit your needs. If you do not exercise, you need to watch your carbohydrate and calorie consumption very carefully. If you do exercise, you can have more carbs in your diet. You can take breaks from the diet and come back on it at any time. In fact, while on the break, you still can use it to your advantage by doing weight lifting exercises to build muscle.

You adjust your level of carbohydrate consumption by varying the proportion of normal-carb to limited-carb days in each week. This is known as a carb cycling regimen. The easiest and most basic cycling regimen is a 1–6 regimen. The first number is your number of normal-carb days; the second, your limited-carb days.

1–1 Cycling Regimen

MON	TUES	WED	THURS	FRI	SAT	SUN
CATABOLISM	ANABOLISM	CATABOLISM	ANABOLISM	CATABOLISM	ANABOLISM	CATABOLISM
LIMITED CARBS	NORMAL	LIMITED	NORMAL	LIMITED	NORMAL	LIMITED

Fat Loss Stages

The diet also offers a subset of carb-control levels, described next. It is an effective way to fine-tune your carb consumption on limited-carb days. As you go through the Carb Cycling Diet stages, the amount of food you eat will gradually decrease but it happens slowly, so you probably will not notice it at first.

Listed below are the three levels:

- Level A (300 grams a day) is the least restrictive. If you eat six meals a day, you can consume about 50 grams of carbs at each meal. (Bear in mind that the normal RDA for carbs ranges from 300 to 400 grams a day.) At Level A, the diet's starting point, you stop eating sugar and all foods containing white flour. Also, no sweet juices are allowed. You'll also learn how to manage those pesky cravings for pleasure foods.
- Level B (200 grams a day). The carb allowance is reduced to about 33 grams of carbs at each of the six meals. In addition, at Level B, you stop eating potatoes and drinking regular milk (2% and 1% milk is allowed). This stage is based on eating whole wheat grain products.
- Level C (100 grams a day) is the advanced and most restrictive stage. You are limited to 16 grams of carbs at each of six meals. You should restrict, but not completely, unrefined carbohydrates.

These stages will bring you to the point when hunger and cravings become tolerable and manageable. The fat loss will be an inevitable result of these changes. The goal of the Carb Cycling Diet is not just to lose weight, a few pounds of fat and muscle. Who wants to look old and skinny? The goal of the diet is to lose fat by increasing the hormonal levels so you can look lean and keep your youthful appearance. If you combine this diet with exercise, you'll have more elastic and vibrant skin, feel energetic and capable of doing physical things that will remind you of your younger days.

Why You Should Count Calories

Few people want to bother with counting calories. But as studies show, those who calculate their daily calorie intake are the most successful in losing fat and keeping fat off. Let me give you some sage advice: do it, especially for these first six weeks. The calculation of calorie balance provides a vital guideline to understanding the metabolic state of your body. If the calorie balance is negative (that is, you have consumed fewer calories than you've burned in catabolism), expect fat loss. If it is equal to your daily calorie requirements, you will not lose fat but but you can count on effective protein metabolism. If the balance is positive (that is, you have consumed more calories than you have burned in—anabolism), you will build muscle but need to make sure you prevent fat gain by exercising before eating. Start a food diary and record the number of calories you consume daily. In two to three months, you will learn the calorie values of various foods and there will no longer be a need to keep a diary or count calories. Soon you will be able to judge your caloric intake based on amount of foods you consume.

Most people err in calorie calculation, and it is almost always on the high side. That gives the user an impression that he or she has a calorie deficit when in reality they do not. Many times my patients tell me, "I use online software to count calories. I eat 1,500 calories a day, and burn 2,000, but don't see fat loss." Several factors play a role here. One of them is the precision of calculation. The technology is evolving but we still rely a century-old formula for calculating the BMR. This old formula allows up to a 13 percent error in calculation. For example, if a boxer and a couch potato are the same age, weight, and height, the old formula gives them the same BMR—but it stands to reason that the boxer has more muscle mass and therefore a higher BMR. When a patient tells me he or she burns 3000 calories a day, I adjust that to about 2700. Many people underestimate the number of calories they eat and overestimate the number they burn doing exercise. While 100 calories worth of miscalculations may not make a difference, a little here and there every day can add up.

The Carb Cycling Diet is, by its nature, a calorie-counting diet. I suggest that you count calories, especially on limited-carb days, for the first six weeks. After that you will learn the food calorie values and be able to estimate the caloric intake without doing precise calculations. Why? Your success depends on it. You'll want to know your target calorie intake, especially on your limited-carb days, in order to get the most out of the diet. Moreover, for effective weight loss you want to be sure that you are in Negative Calorie Balance. To boost metabolism and build protein you want to make sure that you consume at least your Daily Calorie Needs.

CALORIE CYCLING

Carbohydrate cycling is, in essence, a form of calorie cycling. On normal-carb days, you increase calorie intake to your Daily Calorie Needs or above; on limited-carb days, decrease it below your Daily Calorie Needs.

For those who wish to get rid of stubborn fat, I recommend that you continue an introductory regimen (not eating refined carbs on normal-carbs days) beyond six weeks. In this case you are still cycling calories by eating more unrefined carbs on normal-carb days. This type of cycling works well for those who have hard time controlling cravings for sweets. Not eating refined carbs prevents spikes in insulin secretion and thus diminishes hunger and cravings for sweets.

CALCULATING CALORIES

Here's an easy formula to calculate the lowest number of calories you can consume on your limited-carb days. Multiply your current weight in pounds by 8. For example, if your current weight is 198 pounds, the lowest number of calories to consume would be 1584. You should only stick to this low-calorie consumption for short periods of time, no more than 5 days a week. Do not go below weight × 8 number of calories! Your BMR will diminish if you go beyond this number.

To calculate the optimal number of calories to consume on limited-carb days, simply add a zero to your weight. So, a 198-pound man would need 1980 calories. This should be your target amount for long-term usage. Use it most of the time.

For normal-carb days, men should add 1100 calories to the optimal limited-carb number if you do not exercise and 1600 if you exercise. Women should add 700 and 1200 calories correspondingly.

Example for a 198-pound exercising man on a 2–3 regimen:

CARBS	Normal	Normal	Limited	Limited	Limited	Normal	Normal
CALORIES	3580	3580	1980	1980	1980	3580	3580

How to Lose Weight without Exercise

While this diet works best when combined with exercise, you can still benefit from it if you don't exercise. The amount of glycogen stored in the body equals about 200 grams in the muscles and 70 grams in the liver. Muscle glycogen serves as an energy source for muscles and the liver's glycogen is used to maintain blood sugar at normal values.

Liver glycogen is the key to carbohydrate cycling if you choose not to exercise. The liver's glycogen can be depleted—without exercise—by restricting carb intake for one day. During low-carb days the liver's glycogen becomes depleted. It restores on normal-carb days. The amount of glucose that can be stored in liver glycogen is smaller than that in muscle glycogen. So be cautious about the amount of refined carbs you consume. Remember, if you don't exercise, you will have to monitor your refined carb intake more closely.

Your Six-Week Carb Cycling Program

The Carb Cycling Diet is a diet for life. As we learned, you can continually adjust the diet to your goals and your lifestyle. So, the programs presented here are really starting programs to jumpstart your metabolism and get your body accustomed to cycling regimens. Most people prefer Program 1, the more restrictive regimen, since it tends to be easier to control insulin and cravings. However, if you have never dieted before and would prefer to take a slower approach, try Program 2.

Both programs are presented here without an exercise component so that you can focus on getting used to the diet first. However, if you are already familiar with exercise basics and want to start exercising right away, go ahead and take a look at the Carb Cycling Exercise Program in Chapter 8 to see how exercise and diet works together to give you the best results.

You'll notice that there are different regimens for men and women in both programs. It is physiologically more difficult for women to lose fat than men, so women require a greater proportion of limited-carb to normal-carb days.

Here is the Program 1 regimen for women:

Week 1	1–6 cycle, Level A
Week 2	1–6 cycle, Level B
Week 3	1–6 cycle, Level B
Week 4	1–6 cycle, Level C
Week 5	1–6 cycle, Level C
Week 6	1–6 cycle, Level C

Program 1 for men:

Week 1	2–5 cycle, Level A
Week 2	2–5 cycle, Level B
Week 3	2–5 cycle, Level B
Week 4	2–5 cycle, Level C
Week 5	2–5 cycle, Level C
Week 6	2–5 cycle, Level C

Note: Both men and women should avoid refined carbs completely (on both limited- and normal-carb days) for these first six weeks. This helps to lower insulin secretion. On normal-carb days, increase calorie intake by eating all kinds of food except refined carbs. After the sixth week, you can re-introduce refined carbs sparingly on normal-carb days.

During the first week, you will be cutting back on pleasure food. Concentrate on making healthy choices, foods rich in nutrients. During the second week, cut back on the amount of carbohydrates you consume. You still can eat many unprocessed carbohydrates. During the third week, adjust your diet to consume more lean meats, seafood, and low fat milk products. Eat small amounts of unprocessed carbs in small portions throughout the day just to keep your blood sugar from falling too low. When blood sugar falling too low the catabolic hormones are released (cortisol and glucagon).

These hormones bring back lowered blood glucose level by breaking down liver glycogen and protein.

In all six weeks, eat Healthy Breakfast (see the recipe in Chapter 6) and supplement with whey protein if you feel hunger. Your primary goal on limited-carb days should be to create a Negative Calorie Balance by restricting carbohydrate intake.

Here is Program 2 for women:

Week 1	1–1 cycle, Level A
Week 2	1–1 cycle, Level B
Week 3	1–1 cycle, Level C
Week 4	1–2 cycle, Level C
Week 5	1–3 cycle, Level C
Week 6	1–6 cycle, Level C

Program 2 for men:

Week 1	2–2 cycle, Level A
Week 2	2–2 cycle, Level B
Week 3	2–2 cycle, Level C
Week 4	2–3 cycle, Level C
Week 5	2–4 cycle, Level C
Week 6	2–5 cycle, Level C

Note: As with Program 1, both men and women should avoid refined carbs completely for six weeks.

In your first three weeks, you are simply getting used to counting calories and restricting your diet on limited-carb days. Only in Week 4 do you begin to increase the number of limited-carb days to a point where you will begin to see fat loss. This means you will be slower to see results, but it is better to be patient and build up to lasting results than to start too quickly, get frustrated, and quit altogether. If you start on Program 2, find that you adapt quickly to this new way of eating, and would like to progress more quickly, you can go ahead and move to Program 1 at any time.

MANAGING YOUR CARB CYCLING DIET

To manage your diet, keep these six basic rules in a mind:

1. Do not eat refined carbohydrates and fat on the same day. Sweet, fat foods such as cheesecake, regular ice cream, and regular chocolate top the list of the most fattening foods. Sugar-free or fat-free ice cream is better.

2. If you are not exercising, do not drink more than 16 ounces of soda even on normal-carb days. Fructose does not provoke a big insulin spike, because it is able to enter muscle cells and fat cells without the help of insulin, but it is so easily absorbed by your muscle and fat cells that it quickly becomes converted to glucose (unless immediately burned away by exercise) and therefore adds fat. Note that this only applies to artificial fructose such as that found in sodas. Natural fructose, found in most fruits, is fine because fiber slows the rate of fructose absorption.

3. If you are not exercising, avoid maltodextrin, a potent form of sugar found in meal-replacement bars and fat-free food. It is there to replace the fat, but it is a hidden glucose. (The glycemic index of maltodextrin is 105, five points higher than glucose, which is 100.)

4. Do not eat desserts after meals. The sugar will make you hungry soon afterwards and make you crave more refined carbohydrates. This is called "rebound" or "false" hunger. Instead have a fruit.

5. When choosing foods, ask yourself, "Can I burn it off today?" and "What nutrients am I getting from this food?" If you cannot get nutrients from it, the food is not worth eating. Many times we eat because something tastes good, or to comfort ourselves, not because our body needs the nutrients. Consider the nutritional value in a sandwich. Most

white bread gives you empty calories. The small amount of nutrients in a leaf of lettuce and a slice of tomato has little value. Instead, why not eat a salad with sliced chicken breast? Choose foods that are rich in nutrients such as vegetables, soy products, beans, nuts, milk products, instead of those that lacking or low in nutrients, such as pasta, pastry, bagels, or pizza.

6. Do not eat large meals on limited-carb days. Follow the hallowed Japanese rule of hara hachi-bu (stop eating when you are 80 percent full). Become a grazer instead of a glutton. Spread your food consumption throughout the day; eat smaller amounts but more often. Modest portions keep insulin levels steady low. If you have a bowl of oatmeal for breakfast, don't eat it all at once. Instead, eat half of it and snack on the rest between breakfast, lunch, and dinner.

Adjusting the Diet to Your Life

There will be times when you might break your schedule and eat refined carbohydrates when you are not supposed to, for instance. This is not the recommended cycling pattern for fat loss, but every so often you can get away with cheating a bit. After all, could you turn down a piece of your mother's birthday cake? There are two options available: either try to eat more and meet the requirements for a normal-carb day or try to restrict the upcoming food intake and consume less than your Daily Calorie Needs. Your decision should be based on how many carb-restricted days preceded this day. If you had just one carb-restricting day prior to this day then try to restrict upcoming food intake and proceed with aerobic exercise. If you had more than two carb-restricted days, then go ahead, eat more and proceed with strength training exercises.

If you normally exercise but skip it one day, make the day limited-carb, at a restrictive Level C (100 grams of carbs). Stick to protein and green vegetables. That should get you back on track.

A Few Additional Tips

Mark your limited-carb days on a calendar. At the end of the month, count them. If you had at least 20, you can expect results. Keep your cycling schedule on the refrigerator door where you can see the limited-carb and normal-carb days at a glance. A sample schedule can be found at the end of the book or downloaded from www.CyclingDiet.com

Keep in mind:

- Do not start a normal-carb day if you honestly cannot say to yourself, "My previous day was limited-carb and I had a Negative Calorie Balance."
- On limited-carb days, the only way you can lose fat is if you eat fewer calories than your body needs (Negative Calorie Balance).
- Do not become disappointed if you fail to resist cravings. Given time, the hunger and cravings will ease.
- At any time you can switch to calorie cycling with no refined carbs on normal-carb days. Eat more food, including more unrefined carbs, on normal-carb days. This approach helps to achieve ultimate fat loss.
- When eating frequently, be cautious. People tend to consume more calories when they eat more than three times a day. It's a matter of habit. They keep eating the large portions that they are accustomed to. Practice hara hachi-bu (eat to 80 percent full).

If you plan to exercise, start your normal-carb day as a limited-carb day. In another words, do not eat refined carbs until you exercise. Then, if you are unable to hit the gym when you planned, you can just continue as a limited-carb day and try to create a Negative Calorie Balance. This tactic helps to prevent diet failures on the normal-carb days when for some reason you were unable to exercise.

On limited-carb days, eat all the green vegetables you wish.

While there is no limit on fat consumption on limited-carb days, if you want faster fat loss results, limit your fat consumption to no more than 50 grams a day. That's less than two ounces or one-fourth of a cup of fat. Do not restrict yourself on essential oil supplements! (It is only 50 calories a day.)

Do not:

- Starve on low-carb days, i.e. eat less than your weight × 8 calories.
- Overeat on normal-carb days, i.e. eat more than Daily Calorie Needs + 300 Calories.
- Consume excessive amount of fat, i.e. more than 60 grams. (According to U.S. Department of Agriculture the average consumption of fat in 1995 was 101 g for men and 62 g for women.)

Remember to start the Carb Cycling Diet slowly. Do not jump to a high level of calorie restriction. This diet is not meant to be a diet of deprivation. Take your time going through Levels A, B, and C. Do this in the right way, or you might become disappointed if you fail to stick to the regimen and fall short in coping with your craving for refined carbohydrates.

To assure success on limited-carb days, keep a diary and make entries at each meal for the six-week starting program. Avoid temptation by removing from your pantry all refined carbohydrates that you crave. Instead, keep sugar-free snacks available, for example, instant sugar-free chocolate fudge pudding. (Ask your family if they'll support you in this step!)

Let me say a word about alcohol and the diet. Alcohol is a refined carb, and you don't need a personal trainer to tell you what a beer belly is. If you want to have a beautiful body, know what to drink: water, coffee, tea, protein-fruit smoothies and sports energy drinks.

Alcohol tricks your body into conserving fat. Alcohol redirects calories towards fat deposition instead of burning for energy. Even with exercise, if you drink alcoholic beverages, your fat loss can be blocked. So a rib-eye steak and a shot of bourbon provide you with a double whammy. And watch out—alcohol inhibits the production of HGH and testosterone. On normal-carb days, one or two light beers, or a glass of wine, won't do much damage. But do not consume any alcohol on limited-carb days.

Words of Wisdom for Dieters

The instructions given here generally apply to healthy, mature men and women between the ages of 35 and 45: the most dangerous years for weight gain. To avoid damage resulting from severe calorie restriction, you should take action now while you still have a chance. Otherwise, it might become too late. It's not possible to restore lost proteins in the skin or cartilage.

Before undertaking any diet and exercise program, it's wise to see your doctor first. If you are pregnant or have a history of heart problems, have had broken bones, a slipped disc, or some other problem, your family physician can best give you advice based on your medical history. Then chart out a timetable of where you are now, where you would like to be in six months, and what your goal

---

**A Word to the Wise:
Cold Turkey Is Better than Just One Bite**

When it comes to avoiding refined carbs, many of us face the temptation to have just one bite to satisfy a craving. That tactic doesn't work and never will. Here's why. As soon as you eat even a small quantity of refined carbohydrates—a bite of ice cream, a sliver of chocolate cake—your insulin spikes for a few minutes. After the insulin pushes the glucose into your cells, the blood glucose level drops. Crash. This causes your body to crave more refined carbohydrates, making the temptation even harder to resist than before you took your "one bite." As a result, you end up on a roller coaster ride.

---

is for the next year. If you have not exercised for long time, start slowly and gradually increase the amount and intensity of exercise over time.

It's good to monitor your weight every morning. When weight loss stops, then you are at your maintenance level—the point where you neither lose nor gain weight. To lose more fat, increase your physical activity (either increase exercise time or incorporate interval training) or temporarily switch to Level C and a greater number of limited-carb days. That's the way to regulate your weight, enjoy good health, and still have an occasional ice cream cone.

After the Six-Week Carb Cycling Program

After you've completed you initial six-week program, you have several options:

- If you started with Program 1 and prefer not to add exercise to your regimen, stick to a 1–6 regimen on Level B or C. For women, this means you'll just continue with your latest regimen. For men, this means switching to a slightly more restrictive regimen.

- If you have completed Program 1 and would like to see even more impressive results in fat loss and muscle tone, go on to Part 3 to learn about how to add exercise to your regimen to maximize the Carb Cycling Diet's benefits.

The CARB CYCLING DIET

5

Your Six-Week Carb Cycling Meal Plan

The following meal plans are examples of what you might eat on normal carb days and limited carb days for a six-week period. As you'll see, I recommend consuming Healthy Breakfast (see Chapter 6) every day. There is a reason behind it. This recipe was developed to provide a large amount of soluble and insoluble fiber. Many studies showing that a large intake of fiber diminishes C-Reactive protein and may protect against coronary heart disease by lowering blood cholesterol and triglycerides. Also, it stabilizes blood sugar thus keeping cravings away.

On limited-carb days, you should still consume some fat. It's best to consume wholesome fats such as Omega-3, Omega-6, and Omega-9. A great source is fish oil, which you can buy in a health food store. Buy only supplements that have been detoxified. Almost all fish, especially those from fish farms, are contaminated with heavy metals, mercury, and PCBs. That's not good for anybody, especially young people and mothers. A couple good brands are Health from the Sun and Spectrum. You should consume at least 5 grams of healthy fats a day (4 capsules equal to 50 calories). The optimum amount is 10 to 15 grams.

In this chapter, you'll find meal plans for normal-carb days as well as for each level of limited-carb days. This way, you can adjust your meal plans according to whatever regimen is most appropriate for you. Remember, the Carb Cycling Diet is designed to be very flexible, so don't feel you need to follow these meal plans exactly. Also, you'll see that you can always use recipes from a more limited level, if you'd like (a Level C recipe on a Level A day, for instance). Recipes for each level can be found in the next chapter. Just stay within the guidelines outlined in the previous chapter, and you'll see results.

Meals for a Normal-Carb Day

On a normal-carb day, you may eat approximately 350 to 400 grams of carbohydrates. That is the typical amount of carbohydrates in the average adult's daily diet. The ratio of carbs/protein/fat should be 3/2/1. This is when you are regenerating muscle tissue, bone, skin, and cartilage. It's a day when you consume your Daily Calorie Needs or create a Positive Calorie Balance if you are muscle building.

While all carbohydrates are allowed on a normal-carb day, here are some general recommendations. Except within two hours after exercise, do not eat too many refined carbohydrates in one sitting. For those who exercise and concentrate on muscle building, the best time to eat refined carbohydrates is within two hours after you exercise, preferably 4 times every 30 minutes. Those who do not exercise should eat refined carbs for breakfast and try to avoid it in the second half of the day.

Those who want to build muscles should consume some protein along with the refined carbs right after exercise, in a ratio of one part protein to four parts carbohydrate. If you are not exercising, don't overeat refined carbs like cookies, cake, and pie. If you choose to eat these foods, eat them sparingly. When choosing your menu, give first choice to foods that are full of nutrients.

Right here, let's put in a special word for honey. Raw honey from bees is a nutrient-rich product of Mother Nature. Feel free to use three to four teaspoons of honey on your normal-carb days.

Drink Green Tea and Eat More Beans!

As you probably know, the occurrence of cardiovascular diseases, cancer, and diabetes in China and Japan is considerably less than in Western societies. One of the reasons is that people from those areas include large amounts of beans and green tea in their diet. Green tea suppresses the growth of cancer cells, has anti-aging properties, and increases exercise performance. Beans are rich in phytonutrients. The nutritional analysis of beans shows a wide spectrum of bioactive substances such as bioflavonoids, vitamins, minerals, antioxidants, fiber, and amino acids.

Beans are low in fat and high in protein and calcium. Notably, white beans contain an ingredient that helps to prevent digestion and absorption of starches in the blood stream. Beans are a good source of unprocessed carbohydrates and fiber. They provide a supply of long lasting energy to the body. Also, if lightly undercooked, they stimulate bowel movement, which cleans up the digestive tract.

We recommend using beans in salads and as side entries. Please refer to the Recipes section for some examples. Keep in mind that because beans contain so much fiber and nutrients, they are very healthy. Consuming beans can prevent many diseases including gastrointestinal cancer, osteoporosis, and diabetes.

NORMAL-CARB DAY MEAL PLANS

NORMAL-CARB DAY I

(Eat as you normally would, but watch your fat consumption. Between meals, have a fruit snack.)

9 a.m. — Breakfast (540 Cal, Carbs: 91 g)

2 pancakes with jam, or cereal with milk or bagel with cream cheese

Coffee with 1% milk

Noon — First Lunch (460 Cal, Carbs: 53 g)

1 cup vegetable soup

1 cup ice cream

2 p.m. — Second Lunch (380 Cal, Carbs: 71 g)

Pasta with cheese and sauce

6 p.m. — Dinner (780 Cal, Carbs: 47 g)

Steak and fried potatoes

7 p.m. — Snack

Total for Normal-Carb Day 1:   2160 Cal, Carbs: 262 g

NORMAL-CARB DAY 2

9 a.m. — Breakfast (539 Cal, Carbs: 53 g)

Bagel with cream cheese

Coffee with 2% milk

Noon — First Lunch (200 Cal, Carbs: 25 g)

Italian wedding soup

2 p.m. — Second Lunch (438 Cal, Carbs: 65 g)

Slice of pizza

I cup yogurt

6 p.m. — Dinner (780 Cal, Carbs: 47 g)

Steak with mashed potatoes

7 p.m. — Snack (330 Cal, Carbs: 36 g)

Tuna sandwich

Total for Normal-Carb Day 2: 2387 Cal, Carbs: 201 g

NORMAL-CARB DAY 3

9 a.m. — Breakfast (264 Cal, Carbs: 44 g)

I cup of Kellogg's Fruit Harvest Strawberry/
Blueberry cereal with 1% milk

Coffee with 1% milk

Noon — First Lunch (320 Cal, Carbs: 43 g)

Bowl of fruit with fat-free whipped cream

2 p.m. — Second Lunch (911 Cal, Carbs: 144 g)

Pasta with cheese and sauce

6 p.m. — Dinner (938 Cal, Carbs: 30 g)

Turkey breast with boiled broccoli

Low-fat yogurt

Total for Normal-Carb Day 3: 2433 Cal, Carbs: 261 g

Meals for a Level A Limited-Carb Day

Initially at least, limited-carb days will pose the biggest challenge. In the beginning, during what is called Level A, do not eat foods containing sugar or white flour such as candy, cookies, white bread, and bagels. During the first week, your total carbohydrate intake on limited-carb days should be no more than 300 grams a day. That's about 50 grams of carbs during each of six meals. Learn to be a carb counter. Choose unrefined carbohydrates that contain more fiber. The glycemic index will help you to make right choices.

While on Level A, you can eat such foods as fruits, vegetables, beans, rice, and whole wheat pasta, and bread. Maintain this level of eating for the first week to help get over any cravings for refined carbohydrates. Learning to overcome cravings will be the hardest task and will take time.

LEVEL A LIMITED-CARB DAY MEAL PLANS

LEVEL A LIMITED-CARB DAY 1

9 a.m. Breakfast (677 Cal, Carbs: 126 g)

2 cups Healthy Breakfast with blueberries (page 108) (Note: This is a Level C recipe)

Coffee with whole milk and Splenda or Nutrasweet

11 a.m. — Optional Snack

Whey Protein Shake or mix with yogurt (page 109)

Noon — First Lunch (293 Cal, Carbs: 31 g)

1 cup New England Clam Chowder (page 98)

Eggplant Sandwich (page 10)

2 p.m. — Second Lunch (280 Cal, Carbs: 46 g)

1 cup Bean Salad (page 112)

(Note: This is a Level C recipe.)

Japanese (Sencha) green tea (Note: I recommend the Yamamotoyama brand, which is very high quality and tastes very good. If you prefer another brand of green tea, however—including Chinese or other teas—by all means, drink that instead. Besides diminishing hunger, green tea has a long list of health benefits.)

5 p.m. — Optional Snack

Whey Protein Shake or mix with yogurt (page 109)

6 p.m. — Dinner (240 Cal, Carbs: 28 g)

Mozzarella Sandwich (page 100)

Japanese green tea

9 p.m. — Optional Snack

Whey Protein Shake or mix with yogurt (page 109)

**Total for Level A Limited-Carb Day 1 (food only):
1490 Cal, Carbs: 231 g**

Add: + 220 Cal, Carbs +11 g for 1 protein shake

Starve & Binge: The Most Common Mistake

The mistake that people make most often is to starve on limited-carb days and binge on normal-carb days. That defeats the purpose of the Carb Cycling Diet. Make sure you don't feel hunger on limited-carb days. Consume whey protein as much as possible. When you are hungry, eat egg whites (up to 12 a day) and Healthy Breakfast. Eat normally on normal-carb days and stay within your calculated optimal calorie target range. That doesn't mean you can stuff yourself with all those cupcakes you missed on restricted days.

LEVEL A LIMITED-CARB DAY 2

9 a.m. — Breakfast (459 Cal, Carbs: 60 g)

I cup Healthy Breakfast with strawberries (page 108)

I slice whole wheat bread with cream cheese

Japanese green tea

11 a.m. — Optional Snack

Whey Protein Shake or mix with yogurt (page 109)

Noon — First Lunch (350 Cal, Carbs: 58 g)

I cup Brown and Wild Rice Eggplant Salad (page 99)

I whole wheat English muffin

2 p.m. — Second lunch (350 Cal, Carbs: 28 g)

Chicken and Bean Burrito (page 101)

Japanese green tea

5 p.m. — Optional Snack

Whey Protein Shake or mix with yogurt (page 109)

6 p.m. — Dinner (350 Cal, Carbs: 22 g)

Roast Chicken with Potatoes (page 102)

Japanese green tea

9 p.m. — Optional Snack

Whey Protein Shake or mix with yogurt (page 109)

**Total for Level A Limited-Carb Day 2 (food only):
1509 Cal, Carbs: 168 g**

Add: + 220 Cal, Carbs +11 g for 1 protein shake

LEVEL A LIMITED-CARB DAY 3

9 a.m. — Breakfast (288 Cal, Carbs: 48 g)

I cup Healthy Breakfast with nectarines (page 108)

Japanese green tea

11 a.m. — Optional Snack

Whey Protein Shake or mix with yogurt (page 109)

Noon — First Lunch (45 Cal, Carbs: 2 g)

I cup Cucumber Tomato Salad in Sour Cream Sauce (page 105) (Note: This is a Level B recipe)

I whole wheat English muffin   Japanese green tea

2 p.m. — Second lunch (424 Cal, Carbs: 84 g)

Bean Salad (page 112)   2 apples

5 p.m. — Optional Snack

Whey Protein Shake or mix with yogurt (page 109)

6 p.m. — Dinner (319 Cal, Carbs: 18 g)

I Stuffed Tri-Color Pepper (page 121)
(Note: This is a Level C recipe)

I slice whole wheat bread

Japanese green tea

9 p.m. —Snack (209 Cal, Carbs: 54)

2 apples and I orange

Whey Protein Shake or mix with yogurt (page 109)

Total for Level A Limited-Carb Day 3: 1285 Cal, Carbs: 206

Add: + 220 Cal, Carbs +11 g for 1 protein shake

LEVEL A LIMITED-CARB DAY 4

9 a.m. — Breakfast (580 Cal, Carbs: 90 g)

1 cup Healthy Breakfast with apples (page 108)

1 whole wheat English muffin with
2 tbsp peanut butter   Japanese green tea

11 a.m. — Optional Snack

Whey Protein Shake or mix with yogurt (page 109)

Noon — First Lunch (410 Cal, Carbs: 6 g)

230 g Beef Stroganoff (page 118)
(Note: This is a Level C recipe)

2 p.m. — Second lunch (219 Cal, Carbs: 15 g)

1 cup Seafood Salad (page 114)
(Note: This is a Level C recipe)

1 slice whole wheat bread   Japanese green tea

5 p.m. — Optional Snack

Whey Protein Shake or mix with yogurt (page 109)

6 p.m. — Dinner (327 Cal, Carbs: 36 g)

1 slice Pork Chops with Vegetable Mix (page 120)
Japanese green tea

9 p.m. — Snack (144 Cal, Carbs: 38)

2 apples...
Whey Protein Shake or mix with yogurt (page 100)

Total for Level A Limited-Carb Day 4: 1680 Cal, Carbs:

185 **g**

Add: + 220 Cal, Carbs +11 g for 1 protein shake

Meals for a Level B Limited-Carb Day

After one week, it's time to move on to Level B where the restriction extends to regular milk and potatoes. When you become comfortable managing your cravings for sweets, try to reduce your daily consumption of carbs from 300 to 200 grams a day. That's 33 grams of carbs during each of your six meals. It will mean eliminating sugar, white flour products, sweet juice, and potatoes from your limited-carb menu. By the end of the second week, you should be watching your carbohydrate intake more carefully on limited-carb days.

LEVEL B LIMITED-CARB DAY 1

9 a.m. Breakfast (332 Cal, Carbs: 62 g)

1 cup Healthy Breakfast with blueberries (page 108)

Coffee with 2% milk and Splenda or Nutrasweet

11 a.m. — Optional Snack

Whey Protein Shake or mix with yogurt (page 109

Noon — First Lunch (187 Cal, Carbs: 30 g)

Tasty Low-Fat Tuna Sandwich (page 106)

2 p.m. — Second lunch (280 Cal, Carbs: 46 g)

1 cup Bean Salad (page 112)

Japanese green tea

5 p.m. — Optional Snack

Whey Protein Shake or mix with yogurt (page 109)

6 p.m. — Dinner (280 Cal, Carbs: 5 g)

1 cup Scallop and Shrimp Salad (page 113)

Japanese green tea

9 p.m. — Optional Snack

Whey Protein Shake or mix with yogurt (page 109)

Total for Level B Limited-Carb Day 1(food only): 1079 Cal, Carbs: 143 g

Add: + 220 Cal, Carbs +11 g for 1 protein shake

LEVEL B LIMITED-CARB DAY 2

9 a.m. — Breakfast (274 Cal, Carbs: 52 g)

1 cup Healthy Breakfast with strawberries (page 108)

Japanese green tea

11 a.m. — Optional Snack

Whey Protein Shake or mix with yogurt (page 109)

Noon — First Lunch (93 Cal, Carbs: 15 g)

1/2 Tasty Low-Fat Tuna Sandwich (page 106)

2 p.m. — Second lunch (178 Cal, Carbs: 5 g)

150 g Sautéed Chicken with Artichoke Hearts
    and Onions (page 117)

Japanese green tea

5 p.m. — Optional Snack

Whey Protein Shake or mix with yogurt (page 109)

6 p.m. — Dinner (327 Cal, Carbs: 36 g)

1 slice Pork Chops with Vegetable Mix (page 120)

Japanese green tea

9 p.m. — Snack (144 Cal, Carbs: 38 g)

2 apples

Whey Protein Shake or mix with yogurt (page 109)

**Total for Level B Limited-Carb Day 2(food only):
1016 Cal, Carbs: 146 g**

Add: + 220 Cal, Carbs +11 g for 1 protein shake

LEVEL B LIMITED-CARB DAY 3

9 a.m. — Breakfast (288 Cal, Carbs: 48 g)

1 cup Healthy Breakfast with nectarines (page 108)

Japanese green tea

11 a.m. — Optional Snack

Whey Protein Shake or mix with yogurt (page 109)

Noon — First Lunch (135 Cal, Carbs: 7 g)

1 cup Bulgarian Cold Cucumber Soup in Yogurt (page 103)

Japanese green tea

2 p.m. — Second Lunch (280 Cal, Carbs: 46 g)

1 cup Bean Salad (page 112)

5 p.m. — Optional Snack

Whey Protein Shake or mix with yogurt (page 109)

6 p.m. — Dinner (250 Cal, Carbs: 5 g)

1 Stuffed Tri-Color Pepper (page 121)

Japanese green tea

9 p.m. — Snack (144 Cal, Carbs: 38 g)

2 apples

Whey Protein Shake or mix with yogurt (page 109)

Total for Level B Limited-Carb Day 3: 1097 Cal, Carbs: 144 g

Add: + 220 Cal, Carbs +11 g for 1 protein shake

LEVEL B LIMITED-CARB DAY 4

9 a.m. — Breakfast (301 Cal, Carbs: 60 g)

1 cup Healthy Breakfast with apple (page 108)

Japanese green tea

11 a.m. — Optional Snack

Whey Protein Shake or mix with yogurt (page 109)

Noon — First Lunch (189 Cal, Carbs: 13 g)

1 cup French Onion Soup Low-Carb Style (page 104)

2 p.m. — Second Lunch (193 Cal, Carbs: 4 g)

150 g Spanish Style Chicken (page 116)

(Note: This is a Level C recipe)

Japanese green tea

5 p.m. — Optional Snack

Whey Protein Shake or mix with yogurt (page 109)

6 p.m. — Dinner (327 Cal, Carbs: 36 g)

1 slice Pork Chops with Vegetable Mix (page 120)

Japanese green tea

9 p.m. — Snack (144 Cal, Carbs: 38)

2 apples

Whey Protein Shake or mix with yogurt (page 109)

Total for Level B Limited-Carb Day 4: 1154 Cal, Carbs:

151 g

Add: + 220 Cal, Carbs +11 g for 1 protein shake

Meals for a Level C Limited-Carb Day

At Level C, count carbohydrates very closely. One hundred grams of carbohydrates a day is all you can get away with at Level C. Level C is the recommended level for those who do not exercise. The carbohydrates from beans and other vegetables will usually make up your daily allowance. It's largely a matter of meats, fish, chicken, beans, small amounts of Healthy Breakfast (please see recipes section) plus green vegetables and salad.

Your menu on limited-carb days at Level C consists mostly of protein accompanied by greens. Protein will keep you from getting hungry while providing a relatively small amount of calories. Good choices of fat free protein include tuna (canned in water), frozen scallops, shrimps, turkey, white chicken meat (without skin), and lean pork. You will lose fat because you have a Negative Calorie Balance as a result of eating a protein-rich diet. If you eat a lot of fat on this day, you might not lose fat. In this case calories are calories, no matter where they come from. A great way to manage hunger is to boil a dozen eggs. Separate the whites from the yolks and keep the whites in the refrigerator. When hunger strikes, eat some egg whites for a quick pick-me-up.

Some of my patients have cut out all carbs on Level C. That is not desirable. I do not want people to go into a state of ketosis as the Atkins or South Beach diets advocate. I urge people to eat unrefined carbs in small quantities even on Level C—rolled oats (as in Healthy Breakfast), wild rice, beans, or a few slices of whole wheat English muffin.

LEVEL C MEAL PLANS

LEVEL C LIMITED-CARB DAY I

9 a.m. — Breakfast (288 Cal, Carbs: 51 g)

I cup Healthy Breakfast with blueberries (page 108)

Coffee with 2% milk and Splenda or Nutrasweet

11 a.m. — Optional Snack

Whey Protein Shake or mix with yogurt (page 109)

12 p.m. — Lunch (280 Cal, Carbs: 46 g)

I cup Bean Salad (page 112)

Japanese green tea

5 p.m. — Optional Snack

Whey Protein Shake or mix with yogurt (page 109)

6 p.m. — Dinner (185 Cal, Carbs: 3 g)

Spinach and Cheese Omelette (page 111)

Japanese green tea

9 p.m. — Optional Snack

Whey Protein Shake or mix with yogurt (page 109)

**Total for Level C Limited-Carb Day I (food only):
753 Cal, Carbs: 100 g**

Add : + 220 Cal, Carbs +11 g for I protein shake

LEVEL C LIMITED-CARB DAY 2

9 a.m. — Breakfast (274 Cal, Carbs: 52 g)

I cup Healthy Breakfast with strawberries (page 108)

Japanese green tea

11 a.m. — Optional Snack

Whey Protein Shake or mix with yogurt (page 109)

12 p.m. — Lunch (280 Cal, Carbs: 5 g)

I cup Scallop and Shrimp Salad (page 113)

Japanese green tea

5 p.m. — Optional Snack

Whey Protein Shake or mix with yogurt (page 109)

6 p.m. — Dinner (327 Cal, Carbs: 36 g)

I slice Pork Chops with Vegetable Mix (page 120)

Japanese green tea

9 p.m. — Optional Snack

Whey Protein Shake or mix with yogurt (page 109)

**Total for Level C Limited-Carb Day 2 (food only):
881 Cal, Carbs: 93 g**

Add: + 220 Cal, Carbs +11 g for 1 protein shake

LEVEL C LIMITED-CARB DAY 3

9 a.m. — Breakfast (288 Cal, Carbs: 48 g)

1 cup Healthy Breakfast with nectarines (page 108)

Japanese green tea

11 a.m. — Optional Snack

Whey Protein Shake or mix with yogurt (page 109)

Noon — Lunch (193 Cal, Carbs: 4 g)

150 g Spanish Style Chicken (page 116)

Japanese green tea

5 p.m. — Optional Snack

Whey Protein Shake or mix with yogurt (page 109)

6 p.m. — Dinner (250 Cal, Carbs: 5 g)

1 Stuffed Tri-Color Pepper (page 121)

Japanese green tea

9 p.m. — Snack (137 Cal, Carbs: 35)

1 orange and 1 medium apple

Whey Protein Shake or mix with yogurt (page 109)

Total for Level C Limited-Carb Day 3: 868 Cal, Carbs: 92 g

Add: + 220 Cal, Carbs +11 g for 1 protein shake

LEVEL C LIMITED-CARB DAY 4

9 a.m. — Breakfast (301 Cal, Carbs: 60 g)

1 cup Healthy Breakfast with apple (page 108)

Japanese green tea

11 a.m. — Optional Snack

Whey Protein Shake or mix with yogurt (page 109)

Noon — Lunch (410 Cal, Carbs: 6 g)

230 g Beef Stroganoff (page 118)

Japanese green tea

5 p.m. — Optional Snack

Whey Protein Shake or mix with yogurt (page 109)

6 p.m. — Dinner (327 Cal, Carbs: 36 g)

1 slice Pork Chops with Vegetable Mix (page 120)

Japanese green tea

9 p.m. — Optional Snack

Whey Protein Shake or mix with yogurt (page 109)

Total for Level C Limited-Carb Day 4: 1038 Cal, Carbs: 102 g

Add: + 220 Cal, Carbs +11 g for 1 protein shake

Coping with Sweet Cravings

Here are some tips to help you resist cravings on limited-carb days:

- Tell yourself, "I can eat this doughnut tomorrow. Today, I must avoid it."

- Have a whey protein shake. You may drink some anytime during the day. Add it into the cup with your favorite nonfat yogurt. There is no limit to the amount you may have.

- Even if you are not hungry, you should eat every two hours. Eat small amounts of protein—beef, chicken, pork, tofu, or egg whites (up to dozen a day). This will prevent hunger and stop cravings before it hits you. Remember this preventive tactic.

- Have a sugar-free "cheat" snack when a craving hits. These include sugar-free hot chocolate, sugar-free ice cream, and sugar-free chocolate pudding.

- If you cannot resist a craving, eat fruit instead of refined carbohydrates. Fructose from fruit will not cause a chain reaction because it does not call up a spike in insulin secretion.

- To stop your nighttime cravings on a limited-carb day, use supplements. After 6 p.m., use liquid L–Carnitine (2 to 6 tablespoons) or sugar control supplements containing chromium and vanadium to prevent sweet cravings at nighttime. Take them daily for the first two months to help you get accustomed to the new eating pattern.

Given time, you will adjust to the new eating schedule while you learn your weak points and how to prevent cravings. In the end, you will have control over your weight.

The CARB CYCLING DIET

6

Recipes for Limited-Carb Days

As you've seen in the meal plans, the Carb Cycling Diet is very flexible. As long as you stay within the basic guidelines established in Chapter 4 for calories and carbs per day, you can eat pretty much anything you want. The recipes included here are just to get you started. You'll see that I've included more Level C recipes than Level A or B because those are the recipes with which most of my clients need help. Also, because Level C is the most restrictive, you can use those recipes on any day (even on normal-carb days).

Level A Recipes
New England Clam Chowder

3 dozen hard-shell or littleneck clams, each about 3" in diameter, shucked (about 3 cups) with the juices reserved

2 medium boiling potatoes, diced into ½" cubes

5 slices of lean bacon, cut into ¼" squares

1 large onion, finely chopped

2½ cups milk

¾ cup light cream

½ tsp crumbled dried thyme

¾ tsp salt

freshly ground pepper

4 tsp butter

Nutrients
Serving size: 1 cup

Calories	130
Fat	18 g
Carboydrate	13 g
Fiber	1 g

Chop the clams into small pieces, strain 1 cup of their juices, and set both aside. Boil the potatoes in enough water to cover completely till they are soft. Drain, reserving ½ cup of boiling liquid in the saucepan, and set potatoes aside.

In a heavy large saucepan, fry the bacon pieces on high heat till they are browned; remove, leaving the fat in the pan, and set bacon aside. Add onions to the fat and cook on a lower setting until they are translucent and soft. Stir in the reserved clam liquor, reserved water, and the clam pieces. Reduce heat to low, cover, and simmer for 13 minutes.

Meanwhile, in a separate saucepan, warm the milk and cream on medium heat until bubbles appear around edges. Pour into the simmering clam mixture and mix well. Stir in the thyme, salt, pepper, and bacon pieces. Add more salt to taste, if desired. Serve with a teaspoon of butter in each plate.

Makes 4 servings.

Note: According to New Englanders, the clam chowder tastes better if it is cooled to room temperature and reheated once more before serving.

Brown and Wild Rice Eggplant Salad

1 cup of brown and wild rice mix

1 medium eggplant, cut into 1" cubes

1 small red pepper, cut into ¾" squares

1 small green pepper, cut into ¾" squares

1 medium onion, cut into ¾" squares

3–4 garlic cloves, minced

3 tbsp olive oil

1 tsp salt

½ tsp pepper

chopped walnuts, slightly toasted

6–7 medium leeks, cut into ¼" slices

Dressing:

3 tbsp olive oil

juice of 1 lemon

½ tsp salt

¼ tsp pepper

Nutrients	
Serving size: 1 cup	
Calories	210
Fat	5 g
Carboydrate	32 g
Fiber	4 g

Carefully wash and boil rice in 1½ cups of water or according to packaging instructions. Set aside in a large pot or serving bowl.

Preheat oven to 350°F. Place eggplant, red and green peppers, and onion in a 9"x12" glass baking pan. Covered with minced garlic, 3 tbsp olive oil, 1 tsp salt, and ½ tsp pepper. Bake for about 50 minutes. Add to rice.

Prepare dressing by mixing olive oil and lemon juice with salt and pepper. Add dressing, walnuts, and leeks to rice and eggplant mixture. Cool and enjoy served alone or with a meat dish.

Makes 4 servings.

Eggplant Sandwich

1 medium eggplant, cut crosswise into slices

4 tbsp olive oil

6 slices whole wheat bread

½ 1-lb package Biazzo® or other brand part-skim mozzarella, cut into thin slices

6 oil-packed dried tomatoes, drained

1 bunch basil

Nutrients Serving size: 1 slice	
Calories	460
Fat	31 g
Carboydrate	46 g
Fiber	3 g

Preheat broiler. Place eggplant slices on rack in broiling pan. Brush both sides with olive oil. Broil 10 to 12 minutes until browned. Place mozzarella on top of bread slices. Put in broiler for a few minutes until the mozzarella melts. Place basil, dried tomatoes, and eggplant slices on top.

Makes 6 servings.

Mozzarella Sandwich

1 whole wheat English muffin, halved

2 slices (30 g each) of Biazzo® or other brand part-skim mozzarella cheese

1 bunch basil, optional

1 oil-packed dried tomatoes, drained (optional)

Nutrients Serving size: 1 English muffin	
Calories	240
Fat	12 g
Carboydrate	28 g
Fiber	3 g

Slice mozzarella cheese in thin slices. Place on skillet over low heat. Heat until cheese start melting. Toast English muffin halves. Place cheese over muffin. Place basil and dried tomato on top (optional).

Makes 1 serving.

Chicken and Bean Burrito

vegetable cooking oil spray

1 whole boneless chicken breast, sliced

1 sweet red onion, chopped

1 sweet bell pepper, chopped

3 sprigs of parsley, chopped

salt and pepper to taste

1 cup of precooked black beans

1 cup of precooked brown rice

1 whole-wheat wrap

Nutrients
Serving size: 1 burrito

Calories	380
Fat	6 g
Carboydrate	54 g
Fiber	4 g

Spray pan with oil and heat on medium. Sauté chicken, onion, and bell pepper until chicken is browned and cooked through. Add salt and pepper to taste. Place chicken mixture, rice, and beans in whole-wheat wrap. Add parsley.

Makes 1 serving.

Roast Chicken with Potatoes

1 chicken

3-4 fresh sage sprigs, including loose leaves

salt

2 garlic cloves

3–4 fresh thyme sprigs

1 tbsp fresh thyme, chopped

½ tsp paprika

1 tbsp barbeque sauce

4 medium potatoes

Nutrients

Serving size: 1 50 g chicken, 1 medium (100 g) potato

Calories	350
Fat	6 g
Carboydrate	22 g
Fiber	1 g

Preheat oven to 375°F. Place chicken in roasting pan. Place sage leaves under loosened skin of chicken. Place salt, garlic, thyme sprigs, and sage springs inside cavity of chicken. Sprinkle with chopped thyme and paprika. Put 4 potatoes in the pan with chicken. Roast chicken and potatoes for about 1 hour 30 minutes. Take out the potatoes and let stand in oven for another 30 minutes. Brush chicken with barbeque sauce. Serve chicken with roasted potatoes in pan gravy.

Makes 4 servings.

Level B Recipes

Bulgarian Cold Cucumber Soup in Yogurt

6 small cucumbers

2 tsp salt, divided

2½ cups plain reduced-fat yogurt

1 bunch chopped dill

1½ tbsp finely chopped garlic

2 tbsp sunflower or olive oil

Nutrients	
Serving size: 1 cup	
Calories	135
Fat	5 g
Carboydrate	7 g
Fiber	2 g

Peel the cucumbers and slice them in half twice lengthwise. Dice the cucumbers into ¼-inch pieces. Sprinkle evenly with ½ teaspoon of salt. Set aside at room temperature for about 20 minutes, wash them in a sieve, spread on paper towel, and dry.

Combine the diced cucumbers, yogurt, dill, garlic, and the remaining 1½ teaspoons of salt in a deep bowl; mix them thoroughly. Stir in the sunflower or olive oil little at a time. Set aside in the refrigerator until chilled thoroughly.

Before serving, add ½ cup cold water and ½ cup crushed ice cubes.

Makes 5 servings.

French Onion Soup Low-Carb Style

4 tbsp butter

8 to 10 fresh onions, sliced into ¼" slices

1 tsp salt

1 tbsp flour

8 cups of beef stock

six ½"-thick slices of black or wholegrain bread, crusts removed

2 tsp olive oil

1 garlic clove, minced

six ⅛" slices Swiss cheese

Nutrients	
Serving size: 1 cup	
Calories	189
Fat	9 g
Carboydrate	13 g
Fiber	0 g

Melt the butter with oil in a heavy large saucepan. Add onions and salt and cook until they are golden brown over medium heat. Sprinkle 1 tbsp flour over the onions and continue cooking for another 3 minutes. Add beef stock to the pan, bring to boil, reduce heat and simmer for at least 35 minutes.

Meanwhile, preheat the oven to 350°F. Place bread slices on a cookie sheet and bake for 15 minutes. Remove from oven, brush both sides of each slice with olive oil, turn slices around and continue to bake for another 15 minutes. Remove from oven, brush all slices with garlic and set aside.

To serve, pour soup in individual bowls, top with a toasted bread slice and a slice of Swiss cheese. Serve once cheese begins to melt.

Makes 6 servings.

Eggplant Salad

1 medium eggplant
2 medium onions, finely chopped
4 parsley springs, finely chopped
salt and pepper to taste
4 medium leeks (green and white parts), cut into small slices
2 tbsp olive oil, optional

Nutrients	
Serving size: ¾ cup	
Calories	70
Fat	3 g
Carboydrate	5 g
Fiber	1.5 g

Preheat oven to 275°F. Wash the eggplant and bake without oil till soft. Cool. Peel off the skin and discard. Chop the eggplant into half-inch cubes. Add onions, parsley, salt, and pepper, and mix well. Sprinkle with leek and serve. Add olive oil if desired.

Makes 4 servings.

Cucumber Tomato Salad in Sour Cream Sauce

5 tomatoes, diced into ½" cubes
4 small cucumbers, diced into ½" thick cubes
1 large onion, finely chopped
4 tbsp reduced-fat sour cream
salt and pepper to taste
4 dill sprouts, chopped

Nutrients	
Serving size: 1 cup	
Calories	45
Fat	3 g
Carboydrate	2 g
Fiber	0 g

Combine the first 4 ingredients, add salt and pepper little by little to taste, and mix well. Add chopped dill and mix once more to combine. Serve freshly made or chill in the refrigerator up to 4 days.

Makes 5 servings.

Tasty Low-Fat Tuna Sandwich

two 6-oz cans of chunk white tuna in water, drained

1 small onion, finely chopped

4 tbsp fat-free or low-fat sour cream

salt and pepper to taste

4 sprigs of parsley, finely chopped

1 head of iceberg lettuce, finely chopped

2 medium ripe tomatoes, diced

4 slices of Pepperidge Farm German dark wheat whole-grain bread, toasted

Nutrients	
Serving size: 1 sandwich	
Calories	187
Fat	6 g
Carboydrate	30 g
Fiber	4 g

Combine tuna, onion, sour cream, and salt and pepper. Mix well, making sure to squeeze onions with the spoon to extract as much of juice as possible. Add parsley and mix once more. Serve this either on a bed of lettuce and tomatoes for a low-carb meal, or as a sandwich in toasted bread.

Makes 4 servings.

Marinated Aromatized Lamb Kabobs

fresh juice of 2 lemons

½ cup of olive oil

2 tbsp cilantro, finely chopped

1 tbsp garlic, finely chopped

2 tbsp parsley, finely chopped

1 tsp ground ginger

1 tsp ground turmeric

½ tsp ground cumin

1 tsp salt

2 lbs lean boneless lamb, cut into 1" cubes

3 lbs fresh beef suet, cut into 1" cubes

Nutrients	
Serving size: 1/2 skewer (150 g)	
Calories	210
Fat	10 g
Carboydrate	9 g
Fiber	5 g

In a large pot, combine lemon juice, olive oil, cilantro, garlic, parsley, ginger, turmeric, cumin, and salt. Add lamb and beef pieces, toss well to coat, and marinate at room temperature for at least 2 hours.

On 6 metal barbecue skewers, thread the cubes, alternating between lamb and beef pieces. Cook in the broiler 4 inches from the flame for about 15 minutes, turning every 3 to 5 minutes. Remove from broiler. Serve with a side salad or other greens.

Makes 6 servings.

Level C Recipes

Healthy Breakfast

3 cups fat-free milk

1 cup rolled oats, non-instant

⅔ cup organic barley flakes

1 teaspoon flax seed meal (optional)

2 tbsp psyllium husks (whole)

3 packages Splenda (1g each)

pinch of salt

few drops of vanilla extract (optional)

blueberries or other fruit of your choice

Nutrients
Serving size: 1 cup

Calories	249
Fat	0 g
Carboydrate	41 g
Fiber	12 g

Pour milk in a small saucepan, add rolled oats, and bring to a boil. Turn off the flame. Add barley flakes, psyllium husks and flaxseed meal. Add Splenda, salt, and vanilla extract. Mix thoroughly. Serve with blueberries or fruit of your choice.

Makes 3 servings.

Sunday Morning Breakfast

1 cup of nonfat vanilla yogurt (preferably Dannon, due to low sugar content)

½ cup Friendship lowfat cottage cheese (no salt added)

1 cup blueberries, raspberries, or strawberries

light cream, whipped (optional)

Nutrients
Serving size: 1½ cup

Calories	250
Fat	1 g
Carboydrate	25 g
Fiber	0 g

Layer yogurt with cottage cheese in a cup. Spread fruit on top. Add whipped light cream if desired.

Makes 1 serving.

Whey Protein Shake

2 scoops (30 g each) whey protein powder
1 cup berries, any kind
1 packet of Splenda (1 g)

Nutrients
Serving size: 60 g

Calories	220
Fat	0 g
Carboydrate	11 g
Fiber	0 g

Put ingredients into blender with 1 cup cold water and ½ cup of ice and mix for 30 seconds.

Makes 1 serving.

Strawberry Smoothie

1 cup of fat-free plain yogurt (preferably Dannon, due to low sugar content)
1 cup of strawberries
½ cup of orange juice
1 package of Splenda (1 g)

Nutrients
Serving size: 2 cups

Calories	208
Fat	0 g
Carboydrate	32 g
Fiber	0 g

Put ingredients into blender and mix for 30 seconds.

Makes 1 serving.

Breakfast Yogurt Fruit Smoothie

2 cups of non-fat vanilla yogurt (preferably Dannon, due to low sugar content)

1 cup of frozen strawberries

1 cup of frozen blueberries

1 banana

½ tsp vanilla extract

other fruits such as apricot, plum, or peach (seed removed), as desired

Nutrients
Serving size: 1 cup

Calories	200
Fat	3 g
Carboydrate	30 g
Fiber	4 g

Place all ingredients in the blender and pulse for about 45 seconds or until all frozen fruit has been blended. Serve immediately.

Makes 2 servings.

Mushroom and Cheese Scrambled Eggs

vegetable cooking oil spray

½ cup onions, sliced

½ cup of sliced sweet pepper

2 slices of Swiss cheese

4 eggs

½ cup of fresh sliced mushrooms or ½ cup of canned mushrooms

salt to taste

Nutrients
Serving size: 150 g

Calories	396
Fat	23 g
Carboydrate	26 g
Fiber	1 g

Spray pan with vegetable cooking oil and heat on medium flame. Mix onions, sweet pepper, cheese, eggs, and mushrooms in a bowl. Add salt and sauté until cooked.

Makes 2 servings.

Spinach and Cheese Omelette

vegetable cooking oil spray
½ cup of defrosted frozen spinach
2 slices of Swiss cheese
4 eggs
salt to taste

Nutrients Serving size: 150 g	
Calories	380
Fat	23 g
Carboydrate	28 g
Fiber	2 g

Spray pan with vegetable cooking oil and heat on medium flame. Mix spinach, cheese, eggs in a bowl and sauté until cooked. Fold it over.

Makes 2 servings.

Feta Cheese Scrambled Eggs

vegetable oil cooking spray
1 large tomato, sliced
4 eggs
4 oz fat-free feta cheese
salt to taste

Nutrients Serving size: 150 g	
Calories	400
Fat	30 g
Carboydrate	16 g
Fiber	0 g

Spray pan with vegetable cooking oil and heat on medium flame. Sauté slices of tomato in skillet until softened. Add eggs, feta cheese, and salt to the tomatoes. Stir constantly until cooked through.

Makes 2 servings.

Bean Salad

3 cups of assorted dry beans
1 sweet red onion, chopped
1 sweet bell pepper red, chopped
4 sprigs of chopped parsley
1 large broccoli head, chopped
3 tbsp olive oil
½ tsp salt
½ tsp black pepper
3 tbsp lemon juice
3 tbsp raspberry white wine vinegar

Nutrients Serving size: 1 cup	
Calories	280
Fat	5 g
Carboydrate	46 g
Fiber	16 g

Soak beans overnight. Boil beans for 10 to 15 minutes. Add all other ingredients and mix.

Makes 6 servings.

Chicken, Feta Cheese, and Spinach Salad

vegetable oil cooking spray
1 chicken breast, cut into strips
⅓ tsp salt
1 sweet red onion, chopped
1 sweet bell pepper, chopped
½ tsp ground black pepper
3 tbsp white wine vinegar
1 bunch spinach
4 tbsp olive oil
1 cup of feta cheese (4 oz)

Nutrients Serving size: 300 g	
Calories	450
Fat	22 g
Carboydrate	10 g
Fiber	3 g

Spray pan with vegetable cooking oil and heat on medium flame. Fry chicken pieces with salt, stirring frequently, until lightly browned. Remove from heat and place in large bowl. Add bell pepper, onion, vinegar, and spinach to bowl with chicken. Add olive oil, toss to mix. Crumble feta onto salad.

Makes 2 servings.

Scallop and Shrimp Salad

1 lb large shrimp

1 lb sea scallops

3 tsp olive oil

one 6-oz can Goya or other brand marinated artichoke hearts

¼ cup fresh parsley, chopped

1 bunch red leaf lettuce

1 sliced lemon

Nutrients	
Serving size: 1 cup	
Calories	280
Fat	17 g
Carboydrate	5 g
Fiber	1 g

Shell and clean shrimp. Rinse scallops under cold water. Pat shrimp and scallops dry with paper towels. Cut each scallop horizontally in half. Put 3 teaspoons olive oil in skillet over medium heat. Add shrimp and scallops; cook, stirring often, for 5 minutes. Remove from heat, add artichoke hearts with marinade and parsley; toss well. Serve with red leaf lettuce and sliced lemon.

Makes 5 servings.

Seafood Salad

10 medium shrimp, shelled and deveined

1 lb calamari, cleaned and sliced into ¼" rings

6 large clams, scrubbed

10 mussels, bearded and scrubbed

juice and zest of 3 lemons

½ cup of extra virgin olive oil

½ cup parsley, finely chopped

Nutrients
Serving size: 1 cup

Calories	150
Fat	3 g
Carboydrate	2 g
Fiber	0 g

In a medium saucepan, bring ½ gallon water to a boil. Drop in the shrimp, cook for about 3 minutes, and remove from water with a skimmer. Place on a paper towel to drain and set aside. In the same water, drop the calamari rings and cook for another 3 minutes; remove the same way as shrimp. Now add the clams and mussels to the liquid, bring to a boil, fishing out mussels and clams as they open. Discard any pieces that have not opened.

Once cooled, scrape the meat out of the shells and place in a bowl along with the shrimp and calamari. Add the lemon juice and zest, olive oil, and parsley and toss till combined. Let the salad sit at room temperature for about 30 minutes before serving. Garnish with lemon wedges and enjoy.

Makes 4 servings.

Creole Shrimp Stew

½ cup sunflower oil

2 cups of coarsely chopped onions

1 cup coarsely chopped green pepper

1 cup coarsely chopped celery

2 tsp finely chopped garlic

4 cups coarsely chopped canned tomatoes, drained

2 medium-sized bay leaves

1 tbsp paprika

½ tsp cayenne pepper

1 tbsp salt

3 lbs uncooked medium shrimp, shelled and deveined

2 tbsp cornstarch mixed with ¼ cup water

Nutrients	
Serving size: 100 g	
Calories	150
Fat	6 g
Carboydrate	3 g
Fiber	1 g

In a large saucepan, heat oil on moderate heat until hot. Add the onions, green pepper, celery, and garlic and cook for about 5 minutes stirring frequently. Stir in tomatoes, 1 cup water, bay leaves, paprika, cayenne pepper, and salt, and bring to a boil over high heat. Reduce heat to low, stirring occasionally simmer for about 20 to 25 minutes. Stir in the shrimp and continue to simmer for about 5 minutes more, or till shrimp are pink.

Stir in the cornstarch-and-water mixture little by little while combining the mixture. Stir over low heat till mixture thickens. Pick out bay leaves and add more seasoning if needed. Serve with wild and brown rice (optional).

Makes 6 servings.

Spanish Style Chicken

3 lbs chicken, cubed into 2" pieces

salt and pepper to taste

⅓ cup of olive oil

2 large onions, cut into ¼" slices

1 tbsp minced garlic

3 small sweet red or green peppers, cut into ¼" slices

½ cup smoked ham, finely chopped

16 oz can of chopped tomatoes

6 black olives, pitted

6 green olives, pitted

Nutrients	
Serving size: 150 g	
Calories	193
Fat	5 g
Carboydrate	4 g
Fiber	2 g

Wash and pat dry chicken pieces, place in a large pot with salt and pepper, and toss to cover completely. In a heavy skillet heat the oil and brown the chicken a few pieces at a time, making sure not to burn the chicken. Transfer to a plate.

Add onions, garlic, peppers, and ham to the remaining oil in the pan and cook for about 10 minutes over moderate to low heat. Add tomatoes and continue to cook on a higher heat until most liquid has evaporated. Return chicken to skillet and continue to simmer on low heat for another 20 to 25 minutes. Stir in the olives and add more seasoning to taste. Serve with wild and brown rice or by itself.

Makes 4 servings.

Sautéed Chicken with Artichoke Hearts and Onions

3 young artichokes, each about 2″ in diameter

1 lemon cut in half

3 tbsp fresh lemon juice

8–10 tbsp clarified butter

12 peeled white onions, about 1½″ in diameter

3½ lb chicken, cut into 8 bite-size pieces

salt and freshly ground pepper, to taste

Nutrients	
Serving size: 150 g	
Calories	178
Fat	2 g
Carboydrate	5 g
Fiber	1 g

Clean the artichokes by cutting off stems and removing any bottom and bruised leaves. Cut 1 inch off the top of each artichoke and with kitchen scissors remove about ¼ inch of each leaf. Rub each cut area with lemon to prevent discoloring. Slice the artichokes in half and then into quarters, and with a small spoon scrape out the hairy chokes and white/pale purple leaves. Place them in a large sauté pan with enough water to cover completely, and add lemon juice. Cook uncovered for 10 minutes, then set aside to dry completely.

In the same pan melt half of the butter. Cook the onions until they are slightly browned, transfer to a plate. To the butter remaining in pan, place chicken, skin side down and brown over moderate heat. Add more butter if needed. Return onions to the pan, cover tightly, and sauté over low heat for about 25 minutes, or until chicken is tender.

In another pan, melt the remainder of the butter, add artichokes, and sprinkle them with salt and pepper. Cover the pan tightly and cook them over lowest heat for about 15 minutes.

Serve the chicken and artichoke hearts with your favorite vegetable side.

Makes 4 servings.

Baked Salmon

vegetable oil cooking spray

6-oz salmon fillet

5 tbsp reduced-fat sour cream

salt to taste

½ onion, sliced

½ lemon, quartered

Nutrients Serving size: 1 6-oz fillet	
Calories	**400**
Fat	**32 g**
Carboydrate	**9 g**
Fiber	**0 g**

Preheat oven to 300°F. Coat baking pan with vegetable oil cooking spray. Put sour cream and salt over salmon. Place salmon in a baking dish, cover with onions, and bake in oven for 20 to 30 minutes. Serve with quartered lemon.

Makes 1 serving.

Beef Stroganoff

vegetable oil cooking spray

½ lb lean beef loin, cut into ½" strips

salt and pepper to taste

4 tbsp fat-free sour cream

1 small onion, sliced

Nutrients Serving size: 230 g	
Calories	**410**
Fat	**33 g**
Carboydrate	**6 g**
Fiber	**0 g**

Spray pan with oil and heat on medium flame. Place beef in skillet, add salt and black pepper. Stir in sour cream and slices of onion. Saute until beef is just cooked through.

Makes 1 serving.

Poached American Summer Salmon

6–7 lbs salmon, cleaned with the head, tail and bones reserved, washed with cold water

fresh lemon juice of 1 lemon

1 large bay leaf

10 whole black peppercorns

1 tbsp salt

1 package of any low-carb cream sauce, prepared per instructions

8 hard-boiled eggs, chopped into fine pieces

fresh dill sprigs

Nutrients Serving size: 1 lb of salmon	
Calories	275
Fat	11 g
Carboydrate	2 g
Fiber	0 g

Please note: You will also need a dampened cheesecloth to wrap the salmon.

Combine salmon trimmings, water, lemon juice, bay leaf, peppercorns and salt in a 6- to 7-quart stainless steel saucepan. Bring to boil over high heat. Reduce heat and simmer covered for 25 minutes. Strain liquid into a poaching pan with a cover.

Wrap salmon into the dampened cheesecloth, leaving 6 inches on each end for lifting the salmon, tie the ends with a string tightly close to the fish, wrap the ends around the handles on either side of the pan. The salmon should be lifted in the pan, liquid covering the salmon by at least 2 inches. Add more water to the pan if necessary. Place lid on pan, simmer on low heat for at least 30 to 40 minutes or 10 minutes for every 1 inch of thickness.

Prepare sauce and add chopped egg. When salmon is poached, remove it from pan, discard the cheesecloth. With a small knife peel off the skin and scrape any remaining gray fat from the salmon; in the same fashion, peel and scrape the skin from the underside.

Serve on a long boat plate. Sprinkle with dill and present with the sauce in a sauce server.

Makes 6 servings.

Pork Chops with Vegetable Mix

vegetable oil cooking spray

2 lean pork slices (100 g each)

salt and pepper to taste

1 medium onion, sliced in rings

1 package frozen vegetables, defrosted (1 lb)

Nutrients	
Serving size: 1 slice	
Calories	327
Fat	8 g
Carboydrate	37 g
Fiber	12 g

Spray pan with oil and heat on medium flame. Add salt and black pepper on both sides of pork. Place pork on skillet. Add slices of onion. Sauté until pork is just cooked through. Serve with vegetables.

Makes 2 servings.

Stuffed Tri-Color Peppers

½ cup of wild and brown rice

2 tbsp butter

1 large onion, diced

2 lbs lean ground beef

1 egg

1 tsp salt

¾ tsp pepper

2 whole red peppers, stems and seeds removed

2 whole yellow peppers, stems and seeds removed

2 whole green peppers, stems and seeds removed

fat-free or low-fat sour cream

Nutrients	
Serving size: 1 pepper	
Calories	250
Fat	14 g
Carboydrate	5 g
Fiber	4 g

Prepare the rice in a large saucepan. Let cool. Preheat oven to 325°F.

In a heavy skillet, melt the butter and cook onion until translucent and slightly browned. Add the onions, ground beef, egg and salt and pepper to the rice in the saucepan. Combine all ingredients. With a spatula or a large wooden spoon, scoop some of the mixture and fill each of the peppers to the top.

Place the peppers upright in a rectangular 9"x12" baking dish and bake for at least 40 minutes or till top parts are slightly browned. Remove and serve with 1 tablespoon of sour cream on top.

Makes 6 servings.

Quick Family Salsa

6 medium ripe tomatoes, finely diced

4 sprigs of cilantro, finely chopped

1 large onion, finely chopped

juice of 1 lemon or 2 tbsp vinegar

1 can tomato paste

2 garlic cloves, minced

salt and pepper to taste

some Tabasco sauce to taste

some paprika to taste

Nutrients	
Serving size: 4 tbsp	
Calories	35
Fat	1 g
Carboydrate	8 g
Fiber	2 g

Mix all ingredients, let sit in refrigerator for at least 2 hours. Serve with your favorite grilled meat or as a dip.

Makes 10 servings.

Chocolate Fudge Dessert

1 Jell-O Sugar-Free Instant Chocolate Fudge pudding

2 cups fat-free milk

Friendship 1% milkfat cottage cheese

Reddi-wip fat-free dairy whipped topping (optional)

Nutrients	
Serving size: ½ cup	
Calories	80
Fat	0.5 g
Carboydrate	11 g
Fiber	0 g

Prepare pudding according to instruction on the package: Beat pudding mix into milk in bowl and whisk 2 minutes. Pour at once into individual serving dishes. Pudding will be soft and ready to eat within 5 minutes. Add 2 tablespoons cottage cheese in each dish. Add fat-free whipped topping (optional).

Makes 4 servings.

After Exercise Dessert

1 Yoplait fat-free cherry yogurt
1 scoop (30 g) whey protein
½ cup Friendship 1% milkfat cottage cheese
Reddi-wip fat-free dairy whipped topping, optional

Nutrients	
Serving size: 1 cup	
Calories	295
Fat	1 g
Carboydrate	21 g
Fiber	0 g

Put ½ cup of cottage cheese in a bowl. Add 1 scoop of whey protein. Mix thoroughly. Add yogurt on top. Add fat-free whipped topping (optional).

Makes 1 serving.

Exercise

The
CARB CYCLING DIET

The Huge Benefits of Exercise

Anabolic hormones improve memory, mood, energy, sex, and skin. They hasten recovery and tissue repair. The more hormones your blood contains, the better your body works, and the better protection you have from diseases. The incidents or duration of many diseases are less in young age. Why? Because of higher levels of hormones and, as a result, higher production of proteins that leads to faster rate of repair. Many studies have demonstrated that vigorous exercise increases levels of Human Growth Hormone and testosterone in the blood. Not every exercise increases hormonal level. For example, exercise without adequate nutritional support can actually lower anabolic hormones level as in the example with Steve K. in Chapter 2. Consider the anabolic hormones as your body's defensive shield. They protect you against diseases and aging.

The advantage of having high anabolic hormones levels include:
- More energy and endurance
- Better and faster repair
- Faster recovery after exercise

Millions of years of evolution have predisposed us to be physically active. Lack of physical activity is unhealthy and leaves us disease prone. Even a small step is better then none, but start slowly and do it regularly. Impulse exercising is not only ineffective but also dangerous.

Just as important, it has been shown that exercise prevents some forms of cancer (breast and gastrointestinal), improves blood pressure control and the blood lipid profile. It also prevents osteoporosis, stroke, and heart attack. The list goes on.

Here is a summary of medical studies showing the benefits of regular exercise; the stars indicate the strength of the evidence (i.e., greater numbers of studies proving the link) that exercise helps to prevent the corresponding disease.

Results of Studies Investigating the Relationship between Physical Activity or Physical Fitness and Incidences of Selected Chronic Diseases.

DISEASE OR CONDITION	STRENGTH OF EVIDENCE
All-cause mortality	☆
Coronary artery disease	☆
Hypertension	☆
Blood lipid profile change	☆
Obesity	☆
Stroke	☆
Colon cancer	☆
Rectal cancer	No difference
Stomach cancer	No difference
Breast cancer	☆
Prostate cancer	☆
Lung cancer	☆
Pancreatic cancer	No difference
Type 2 diabetes	☆
Osteoarthritis	No difference

Adapted from ACSM's *Guidelines for Exercise Testing and Prescription, Sixth Edition*, 2000, Lippincott, Williams & Wilkins. Originally printed in Blair SN. Physical activity, physical fitness, and health. *Res Q Exerc Sport* 1993. 64:365-376.

Aerobic versus Anaerobic Exercise

Many people take the wrong tactic when exercising. In attempt to lose fat and build muscle they cut down on calories and do weight lifting or resistance machines in the gym. They think that they can kill two birds with one stone--build some muscle and burn fat at the same time. What is wrong with this approach? As you've learned in this book you cannot achieve both goals on the same day. Instead, when going to the gym, have a plan for the day: either build muscle or burn fat. How to decide? Your decision should be based on your calorie intake for this particular day. If it's a limited-carb day, proceed with aerobic exercise. If it's a normal-carb day, proceed with anaerobic strength training exercise. The following diagram illustrates the relationship between diet and exercise.

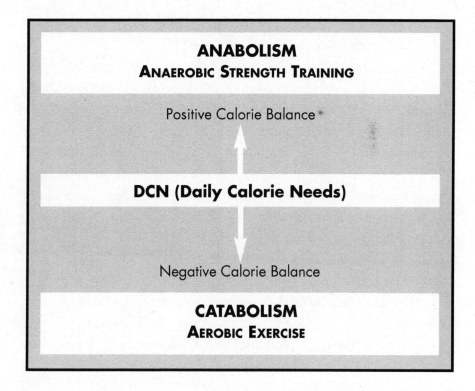

AEROBIC EXERCISE

The process of energy generation can be either aerobic (using oxygen) or anaerobic (without oxygen). Aerobic refers to oxygen available to the muscles for generating energy. Examples of aerobic exercises are running, swimming, rowing, and cycling, where the muscular intensity is not extremely high. Aerobic exercise is typically associated with cardiovascular activities that work the heart and lungs, but strength training can become aerobic if performed with light or medium weights, as in circuit training. Any exercise performed at less then 75 percent of maximum effort is considered as aerobic.

The benefits of aerobic exercise include:
- Increasing tissue sensitivity to insulin
- Burning a large percentage of fat for energy
- Strengthening the heart and lungs
- Improving blood circulation, which delivers more oxygen and nutrients to every cell in your body

The continuous nature of aerobic training will keep your heart rate and oxygen consumption high throughout the workout. Your breathing rate is increased, so the muscles keep burning oxygen. For that reason, you may want to take Co-enzyme Q-10 or NADH supplements before you begin your aerobic workout. These powerful anti-oxidants will combat the oxygen radicals in your blood that forms because of increased oxygen turnover. We'll learn more about these supplements in Chapter 10. There is no need to take both. One of them is enough.

ANAEROBIC EXERCISE

The anaerobic production of energy comes into play in emergency situations when a large amount of energy is needed quickly. Any exercise performed at high intensity (close to maximum effort) would be considered anaerobic.

When we speak of anaerobic exercises, most people think of weight lifting because this type of exercise involves great bursts of power where the energy need is extreme. Not every weight lifting exercise is anaerobic, however. Weight lifting with light weights, as you do in circuit training, utilizes a large percentage of oxygen and does not invoke the release of anabolic hormones associated with anaerobic exercise. To make weight lifting exercise anaerobic you need to pick up heavier weights—more than 50 percent of your 1-RM (the greatest weight you can lift once).

I recommend performing strength training anaerobically, which means using high resistance or heavy weights. However, as we've seen, running and other cardiovascular exercises can also be anaerobic if it is performed at a sufficiently intense level—for example, during a last-minute, full-speed sprint for the finish.

The benefits of anaerobic exercise include:
- A long post-workout calorie-burning effect
- A large amount of lactic acid production, a natural antioxidant
- Body conditioning to improve speed and strength
- The stimulation of Human Growth Hormone, DHEA, and testosterone release, producing anti-aging and health protecting benefits
- The depletion of muscle glycogen, which is very important
- Efficient burning of a large amount of calories in the least amount of time, allowing you to cut exercise time

Strength training builds muscle. The presence of muscle increases your metabolism (BMR) so you can begin to burn more energy even while sleeping. It is also increases your glycogen depot size. That means more glucose from the blood can be deposited in muscles as glycogen instead of going into fat cells. Strength training is essential for lasting fat loss. Muscle is also what gives you energy, better posture, and balance.

The advantage of having more muscles:

- Increase in basal metabolic rate. Muscles are very metabolically active. That means they burn a lot of calories even at rest. Building muscles makes it easier to lose fat.
- Increase in energy and stamina.
- Reassurance of being active and mobile during your retirement years. A review of nursing homes found that more than half of the residents are unable to stand up from the toilet seat without assistance because of atrophied hip muscles. In order to avoid being debilitated by atrophied muscles, you need to take a few steps now. Start weight lifting or strength training exercises and do them regularly.

Many people ask me if they should use exercise machines or free weights. Exercises performed with free weights usually involve more muscles, as you need to maintain balance and stabilize your whole body while performing the exercise. Since more muscles are involved it puts more stress on the body and it reacts with releasing anabolic hormones. However, some muscles are very hard to work out with free weights. They can be better targeted with a machine. The machines are also usually safer to use, especially for beginners who may not know the proper form for each exercise.

Interval and Circuit Training

Both aerobic and anaerobic exercise are important for total-body fitness; aerobic exercise, as we've seen, focuses on burning fat, while anaerobic exercise primarily builds muscle. But in today's fast-paced world, who has time for five aerobic workouts and three anaerobic workouts in one week? Plus, what do you do if you can't bear to give up your daily run or you just can't stand those dreaded cardio machines? Turn your favorite exercise into either an aerobic or anaerobic exercise to suit your needs.

INTERVAL TRAINING

Interval training can be used by anyone as a tool to improve endurance and fitness level. Novices can use it with smaller increments in speed and longer rest intervals. Advanced exercisers can use it to build a better physical shape. In this book I describe methods on how novices can use it with small increments of speed and intensity (Slow-Fast training). Until you reach a high intensity levels this form of exercising will be considered as aerobic exercise. Later, when your fitness level increases and you start using higher speeds and intensity the interval training will become anaerobic exercise.

Interval training is a tool often used by professional athletes in their training routines. It helps them to improve speed and endurance. In this book, I will teach you how to use a modified form of interval training designed for fat loss, general fitness, and good health. Interval training can be performed while walking, running, cycling, swimming, or using gym equipment such as an elliptical machine. Interval training consists of repetitions of exercise and intervals of relative rest. The interval is the relative rest, which to a runner can mean slowing down from a flat-out run to a walk. The repetition is the high-intensity exercise portion of the cycle, followed by the interval of rest.

For those new to interval training, here's a simplified explanation. Let's suppose you can run for 25 minutes before giving out. What if you divided that 25-minute run into runs of eight minutes? That should equal three runs of eight minutes. But if you rest for just a few seconds between each run, you can complete four runs instead of just three. In time, by reducing the three rest periods into two and then one, you will eventually able to run for 32 minutes without stopping. That is the power of interval training. This works for every kind of aerobic exercise.

When it comes to interval training, the main rule to remember is that benefits will accrue only when you get tired and sweaty, not when the workout is easy. One of the main goals of a successful exercise program is to challenge your body by changing the intensity of exercise during the week from low to high. Then the body has a chance to recuperate when the intensity level is low. To begin your interval training, start with Slow–Fast training. Have you ever driven a car with manual transmission? Slow–Fast training is like switching gears while driving in the city. It is a form of interval training but instead of complete stops for rest, you slow down and continue to run at a slower speed. The slow interval should be twice as long as the fast interval. If you are a walker, increase your walking speed a little for two minutes, then slow down for four minutes, then speed up again for two. Same thing for running, cycling, or any other kind of exercise. Do not go for longer fast intervals in the beginning of your program.

Before you proceed to a very high intensity (i.e., very tired and sweaty), you need to become a regular exerciser. That means you're doing three to four days a week of 30 minutes continuous aerobic activity for at least four months. Once you've reached this level, try the following regimen: an intense exercise interval for two minutes followed by no more than two minutes slower rest interval. Those who are already experienced exercisers can start with this regimen immediately. As you gain experience and stamina, the shorter the rest time the greater the benefit. The speed of the intense exercise repetition can vary from 60 to 90 percent of MAX (explained more in Chapter 10) effort.

CIRCUIT TRAINING

Circuit training simply means that you perform different strength training exercises in a sequence, or circuit. Circuit training aims for endurance, but the workouts are short (no more than 50 minutes) so you can complete the prescribed circuit and still make it to work on time. When you first begin circuit training, you will be moving slowly to ensure that you get the form right with each exercise. At this stage, circuit training should be performed on normal-carb days.

At an advanced level, however, you can move quickly from one exercise to the next, shorten your rest intervals, and stick to low-to-medium weights (so as not to overemphasize the muscle-building aspect), thus turning circuit training into an effective aerobic exercise that trains the cardiovascular system. Pay attention to your heart rate. It is important not to let your heart rate slow down during the circuit. At this level, circuit training should be performed on limited-carb days.

Whether you use free weights or gym exercise equipment, the extension phase of each repetition should be performed under tension. If, you do a chest fly, for example, do not relax your muscles and let gravity bring the weight to the original (relaxed) position. Instead, lower it, slowly, within 4 seconds, under the control of your muscles. Bring the weight to one step above the starting position and start another repetition. Your arm should not go to the complete extension. At no point should you allow your muscles to relax.

Keeping these muscles under constant tension produces the maximum glycogen burning effect. New blood can't enter muscles when the vessels are flattened by the tension of surrounding muscle. That denial of oxygen means the muscle is forced to consume local glycogen as its energy source. During your exercise, if you feel a burning sensation in your muscles, that means the glycogen is breaking down into lactic acid, a good sign.

One of the nice things about circuit training is that it is self-calibrating. When you are introduced to a resistance machine, warm-up first with low weight, then set the weight level as high as you think you can lift. Keep adjusting it until you arrive at the greatest all-out weight you can lift—once but not twice. That is known as your one-repetition maximum (1-RM) value. Now set the weight on the resistance machine to 40 percent of your 1-RM. If your 1-RM is 100 pounds, set the weight at 40 pounds. Now you are ready to start. That measurement tailors the resistance precisely to your body. And surprisingly, it is less strenuous than you might expect.

Before you start your circuit, always warm up with five minutes of jogging or cycling. Do some stretching. You could then do three sets of 15 repetitions of each exercise. Another way to organize it is to do three circuits of fifteen repetitions around the gym and you're ready for the showers, all in less than an hour.

Don't be intimidated by the equipment in the gym. In one gym, the exercises might include bench presses, inclined sit-ups, leg presses, lat pulls, back arches, shoulder presses, leg extensions, arm curls, leg flexions, and upright rows. In another, you might face squats, shoulder presses, knee flexions, bench presses, leg presses, elbow flexions, back hyperextensions, elbow-extensions, sit-ups and vertical flies. If you don't know what these machines are for, ask a trainer to show you each machine and demonstrate how it works. This avoids injury and helps you get the most out of your workout.

Incorporating Exercise into the Carb Cycling Diet

Why emphasize the importance of exercise? Because it is the only way to stay fit, energetic, and disease-free. It's the best way to add 10 to 20 quality years to your life. If you calculate the time you spend exercising, it should nearly equal the time you add to your life.

The reason some people don't exercise is because they don't have the time, but I'm not talking about an exercise program so time-consuming that it would violate the labor-standards act. Begin with as little as 15 to 20 minutes a day. Then you can eventually work up to an hour or more if you want to. Start with low-intensity exercises. Then incorporate high-intensity exercise, which boosts anabolic hormone production and provides anti-aging benefits. But remember your body is highly adaptive. It can adjust to exercise and eventually find a way to conserve energy. That is why so many people exercise and get no significant results.

So what's the solution? Fool your body. Change your physical activities. Change the weight and number of repetitions you do. Decrease the number of repetitions and increase the weight. Three to four repetitions with weight close to your 1-RM is better then a few dozens of repetitions with medium weight. The first one increases strength and muscle mass. The last one might have no effect except burning calories. You should alternate aerobic exercise with resistance training like weight lifting or working out with gym equipment. You can incorporate one day of each week's interval training into your schedule. Make sure you have one or two days of complete rest in your schedule. An overtired body will put brakes on all your efforts.

Which type of exercise—aerobic or anaerobic—should you do to lose the most fat? In the beginning, you need to keep two points in mind:

1. The amount and frequency of the exercise you get.
2. The number of calories burned during the exercise (which corresponds to exercise time).

Each type of exercise has its own benefits. The best course of action would be to do both aerobic and anaerobic exercises, cycling them as you do your diet. It is important to find the right balance between the amount of weight lifting and aerobic exercises in your program. This factor is individual to each person and varies with age, sex, body type, etc.

As you age, your level of anabolic hormones decline. That means that, over the years, you need to gradually increase the amount of anaerobic exercise you do and decrease the amount of aerobic exercise in your fitness program. That reassures that you will keep the muscles and your body will produce more anabolic hormones when its production naturally ceases.

THE IMPORTANCE OF HIGH-INTENSITY WORKOUTS

Studies of athletes have shown that the more intense the exercise, the longer the post-workout impact on metabolism and calorie burning. In other words, after intense exercise, you continue to burn calories at an accelerated rate for several hours. A slow-moving workout will burn fewer calories and won't have much of an impact on your post-workout metabolism. Also, intensive weight lifting has a greater impact on post-workout calorie burn than aerobic exercise.

Intensity in a workout puts stress on your muscles and your whole body. The amount of work your muscles perform in a minute depends on the intensity level. In running, it correlates with your running speed. When you lift weights, the heavier the weights, the greater the intensity. That translates as more physical stress on your body. In response, the stressed body releases Human Growth Hormone, DHEA, and testosterone. Low intensity exercises do not produce this beneficial effect and have no anti-aging benefits.

Twenty minutes of intense exercise can deplete your muscle glycogen level to where the fat-producing refined carbohydrates you consume afterwards will not deposit glucose in fat cells. Instead, it will be converted to glycogen. Your goal should be to achieve a higher intensity level over the time. But remember, start easy and slow. Gradually over a period of months, work your way up to a high intensity level. Low intensity, longer workouts should be your basis. Have one high intensity interval training a week. Because only high intensity exercise releases anabolic hormones and gives you anti-aging benefits, you might be tempted to do more than one. But high intensity workouts, by their very nature, can easily lead to overtraining, which brings its own set of health problems. So stick to just one high intensity workout a week.

If your goal is to build muscles, you should follow this basic principle of weight lifting: The optimum workout time for weight lifting is 55 to 75 minutes. To build muscles, you need to achieve the following:

- A level of muscle stress that tears the myofibrils. Myofibrils are components of muscle cells that responsible for contraction. The microtrauma of myofibrils leads to local release of growth factors that stimulate muscle cell to adapt. In response, the muscle cell starts to produce more proteins to repair damaged myofibrils. This is one of the many processes that lead to increase in muscle size.
- A high level of desirable anabolic hormones in the blood. The MAX effort exercises we'll introduce later in the chapter will help to release anabolic hormones.
- An abundance of amino acids and other nutrients.
- A Positive Calorie Balance, about 300 calories more than your Daily Calorie Needs.

To tear muscle myofibrils a certain level of physical stress must be placed on the muscle. When you are young, you can easily reach and tolerate this kind of intensity in a workout. But as you age, it is harder to reach that level. You tire more easily than you did at age 20.

What can you do to raise the intensity to higher levels? Here is a training schedule that can help raise intensity:

5 sets × 10 reps at 70% of 1-RM per workout for four weeks,
4 sets × 8 reps at 75% of 1-RM for the next four weeks,
4 sets × 6 reps at 80% of 1-RM for another four weeks,
then 3 sets × 4 reps at 85% of 1-RM over the final month.

As you can see from this example, the volume of exercise is decreasing over the course of four months but the intensity is rising. This rule applies even to a single exercise session: When intensity is high, the exercise time should diminish. When intensity is low, the exercise time should increase.

To make sure that myofibrils are damaged, make sure that the last 2 sets are performed to the point of muscular failure, no matter how many repetitions it takes. You can also use energy-increasing and stimulating agents immediately before workouts. For details, see the Sports Supplements section.

EXERCISE AND CARBOHYDRATE RESTRICTION

Exercise and carbohydrate restriction go hand in hand. If you want to eat more of your favorite refined carbohydrates, add more exercise to the Carb Cycling Diet. The level of carb restriction depends on your activity level. If you do not exercise, follow Level C for the most of the time. If you exercise regularly at medium intensity, stay at Level B. If you exercise often at high intensity, you can stick to Level A. So, the more frequent and intense your exercise, the more carbohydrates you can eat.

INCORPORATING A CHANGE OF PACE

Exercise, like everything else, can become a boring routine. This is especially true if the same workout routine is performed day after day. You can make your workouts interesting by alternating. Imagine you are a triathlete. On limited-carb days, you can alternate walking, running, biking, and swimming, if you wish. But always keep one important point in mind: You must progress in intensity and work up to a climax. On one or two days of the week, you should push yourself to the limit.

For instance, when performing interval training, play around with different regimens by changing repetition time from 30 seconds to three minutes or rest interval time from two minutes to one minute. See how your body reacts to the change. Do long repetitions one session and short repetitions the next. The Slow–Fast regimen, if performed at high speed, requires a high level of fitness and can be included in exercise routine of advanced exercisers. Beginners can use it but only with small increments of speed.

For interval training, you should put in no more than two hard training days per week with 48 hours of active-recovery time in between. Active-recovery time means a non-intense form of aerobic exercise such as jogging, swimming, or bicycling.

No matter what type of training you do, never become comfortable with your regimen. Always change the repetition and rest interval time. Always challenge your body!

TAKING TIME OFF FROM EXERCISE

Sometimes you may feel tired, suffer from low energy, or have lost your inspiration for exercise. It's a time for a break. Take a week off from any exercise. Let your body recover completely. When you feel fresh and filled with pep and vinegar, return to your workout routine.

With that said, stopping for too long isn't good either. Studies have been conducted to investigate the consequences of a reduced exercise program or a cessation of cardiorespiratory fitness training.

A significant reduction of cardiovascular fitness occurs within two weeks of stopping. Most of the reduction occurs when the intensity of training is reduced. In contrast, decreasing the frequency or duration of daily training had little influence—provided that the intensity was maintained. In other words, intensity is again the key word here. One brisk workout each week helps to maintain the fitness.

Weight Lifting for Women

Some women avoid weight lifting for fear of building muscles that are too big. In actuality, this rarely happens. Successful muscle building requires that high levels of anabolic hormones (testosterone) be circulating in the blood. Since women have lower levels of testosterone, it's much harder to build bulging muscles.

After weight-lifting exercises, you may notice an increase in muscle size. The slight increase in muscle size is attributable to three things: better blood flow, water retention and the plumping effect of muscle glycogen. These changes are not permanent. A few days after you stop weight lifting, the plumping will disappear. If you gain more muscle than you would like, just add more limited–carb days.

But in fact, building muscle has more advantages than disadvantages. It increases your BMR, thus making it easier to drop fat. In another words, muscles will consume so many calories that you will be able to eat more without depositing fat. It increases your energy level and stamina. It makes you stronger and prevents disability later in your life. It makes bones stronger and prevents osteoporosis. Finally, it increases anabolic hormone secretion. So don't be afraid to lift weights!

MAINTAINING ENERGY DURING EXERCISE

There may be times when you need a pre-exercise carb boost. Research shows that carb restriction before exercise is associated with early onset of fatigue during physical exercise. To overcome this effect eat a moderate amount of unprocessed carbohydrates one hour before exercise session.

During exercise, you may consume fructose and caffeine in the form of sports drinks. That should provide a jolt needed to keep going through a workout. (One such drink is called Extreme Energy Shot made by Arizona.) I recommend a small amount of fructose because it provides energy without provoking a large insulin secretion. Studies have shown that insulin blocks the exercise–induced release of Human Growth Hormone. A sports drink will give you sufficient energy to boost exercise intensity and burn 800 calories during a hard workout.

Risks Associated with Vigorous Exercise

You are responsible for yourself. Take care of your body and exercise carefully. If you have reached middle age, begin slowly. Before you start, consult your physician or cardiologist and opthamologist to get a medical clearance. Six months later, do a follow-up with your doctor. For the first year you need to pre-condition your body by low-intensity training and circuit training with one- to two-minute rests. Only then can you take up high-intensity training. The risk of both cardiovascular and orthopedic injuries increases at higher intensities of physical exertion. Increased demands for oxygen during exercise may precipitate complications in a person with heart disease. Sedentary people who engage in sporadic high-intensity exercise, couch potatoes who become roaring Tarzans on weekends, are especially at risk. To prevent these injuries, precede every exercise session with properly performed warm-up and stretching sessions.

Even if you feel fine, you need to get a green light from your family doctor to ensure that your body is able to withstand the high intensity of a vigorous workout. Your doctor may want you to take an X-ray and maybe an electrocardiogram to rule out any possibility of silent cardiovascular diseases (aneurysm, arrhythmias, myocardial ischemia, heart failure, heart valve diseases, etc). In some cases, depending on your age and physical condition, it is the better part of valor to proceed with a more rigorous stress evaluation to make sure that your heart is able to pump blood effectively at high rates (stress test). Many times dangerous conditions lurk beneath the surface until your body is stressed. Once your doctor gives you the thumbs up to vigorous exercise, you can proceed at a cautious rate to begin your exercise program.

Age is not a barrier that should stop you from exercising. For instance, exercise guru Jack LaLanne amazed people with his athletic prowess into his 90s. But when anyone gets older, it becomes harder to engage in high-intensity exercise. And it is certainly more difficult to start an exercise program. The joints have become stiffer. That means losing the full range of motion and flexibility you used to have. Muscles lose their strength too. Consider the following points of advice:

1. Stretch your muscles gently and thoroughly before and after the exercise.
2. Increase the warm-up time to 15 to 20 minutes.
3. Take your joint support formulas regularly.
4. You may need to include additional rest days in your program. Your body usually will tell you when you need a rest.
5. Take a dose of baby aspirin (81 mg) at least once a week.
6. Stop exercising immediately if you feel pain or discomfort in your left arm, jaw, chest, back, or any shortness of breath,

changes in vision, or faintness. Call your doctor promptly for a physical evaluation.

7. Consult your doctor if a joint pain occurs only on one side or does not subside after three days.

Don't engage in high intensity and MAX effort exercise if you have history of:

• High blood pressure
• History of heart attack or stroke
• Any heart conditions
• Aneurysm of aorta or other vessels
• Eye conditions, except astigmatism, near- or far-vision.
• Blood and vessel disorders (phlebitis, arteriosclerosis, etc.)

AGE AND AEROBIC EXERCISE

Because of naturally higher level of anabolic hormones, young people react faster to calorie restriction by losing fat. They recover faster, build muscles faster, and are able to maintain the results longer. For them, running is the best way to exercise aerobically on limited-carb days. That is not true for those who are over 40. After 40, cartilage injury and overtraining becoming major concerns. Solution? If you are over 40 make sure that you have enough rest days in your program, and use the elliptical machine and circuit training instead of running.

The CARB CYCLING DIET

Your Six-Week Carb Cycling Exercise Program

By now, you know all about alternating anabolism and catabolism in order to maximize your fat loss and muscle building and you've seen how you can control both mechanisms to your advantage through diet and exercise. Now it's time to put the two together.

For those who are just starting an exercise program—that is, you have never exercised regularly before, or you haven't been for the past year or more—I recommend that you start with circuit training on normal-carb days and low-intensity aerobic exercises, such as walking with dumbbells, on limited-carb days. For example:

Beginners

	MON	TUES	WED	THURS	FRI	SAT	SUN
EXERCISE	CIRCUIT TRAINING	OFF	WALKING W/DUMBBELLS 60 MINUTES	WALKING W/DUMBBELLS 60 MINUTES	WALKING W/DUMBBELLS 60 MINUTES	OFF	CIRCUIT TRAINING
DIET	NORMAL	LIMITED	LIMITED	LIMITED	LIMITED	LIMITED	NORMAL
GOAL	ANABOLISM	CATABOLISM	CATABOLISM	CATABOLISM	CATABOLISM	CATABOLISM	ANABOLISM

Those who are in intermediate group (exercising regularly for at least four months) should do circuit training on limited-carb days—

by this point, you should be able to do the circuits quickly enough with short rest periods to make it an effective aerobic exercise. (You can also do other aerobic exercises on your limited-carb days.) Regular weight training (not in circuits) should still be done on normal-carb days. For example:

Intermediate

	MON	TUES	WED	THURS	FRI	SAT	SUN
EXERCISE	WEIGHT TRAINING	OFF	AEROBIC EXERCISE	CIRCUIT TRAINING	OFF	AEROBIC EXERCISE	WEIGHT TRAINING
DIET	NORMAL	LIMITED	LIMITED	LIMITED	LIMITED	LIMITED	NORMAL
GOAL	ANABOLISM	CATABOLISM	CATABOLISM	CATABOLISM	CATABOLISM	CATABOLISM	ANABOLISM

Advanced exercisers (regularly exercising for more than a year) should incorporate high intensity interval training (HIIT) into their programs. Remember, by this stage, your intervals should be intense enough and close enough together that they become anaerobic exercise, and can be done either on normal-carb or limited-carb days. (Since circuit training does build muscle, but is not as effective as more intensive weight training, it can be done on either normal-carb or limited-carb days.) For example:

Advanced

	MON	TUES	WED	THURS	FRI	SAT	SUN
EXERCISE	WEIGHT TRAINING	OFF	RUNNING	CIRCUIT TRAINING	OFF	WEIGHT TRAINING	ELLIPTICAL MACHINE INTERVAL TRAINING 20 MINUTES
DIET	NORMAL	LIMITED	LIMITED	LIMITED	LIMITED	NORMAL	NORMAL
GOAL	ANABOLISM	CATABOLISM	CATABOLISM	CATABOLISM	CATABOLISM	ANABOLISM	ANABOLISM

Please note that there is no one uniform regimen that fits everyone. In this chapter, I'll present a 6-week program to help beginners add exercise to your Carb Cycling Diet. But, depending on your age, sex, genetic factors, health conditions, the amount and type of exercise you do, and your goals, regimens need to be adjusted. Once you're comfortable with the different types of exercise, you'll want to experiment with different cycling regimens to find the one that suits you best.

Your Six-Week Carb Cycling Exercise Program

This program is designed to complement Program 1 of the Six-Week Carb Cycling Diet outlined in Chapter 4. If you chose to start with the diet only, you'll see that the carb cycling regimens here are exactly the same as the ones you are used to; you are simply adding exercise to your program. If you are already familiar with exercise basics, you can start here with both the diet and exercise. The exercise program is designed for beginners, though, so don't worry if you haven't been to a gym in a long time.

Remember, you'll see that there are different carb-cycling regimens for men and women. However, you'll see that the exercise program for men and women is very similar. For instance, in both programs, you start by adding low intensity walking to your limited-carb days and circuit training to your normal-carb days. But because the women's regimen has fewer normal-carb days than the men's, women will do fewer circuit-training sessions than men.

Here is the Six-Week Carb Cycling Exercise Program 1 for women:

Week 1   1–6 cycle, Level A. Start with 40 minutes low-intensity walking on limited-carb days and 45 minutes circuit training on normal-carb days.

Week 2   1–6 cycle, Level B. Continue to exercise as in week 1.

Week 3   1–6 cycle, Level B. Increase intensity of circuit training by increasing weight.

Week 4   1–6 cycle, Level C. Incorporate one day of slow-fast interval training on the elliptical machine on limited-carb days.

Week 5   1–6 cycle, Level C. Continue to exercise as in week 4.

Week 6   1–6 cycle, Level C. Continue to exercise as in week 4.

Now, the Six-Week Carb Cycling Exercise Program 1 for men:

Week 1   2–5 cycle, Level A. Start with 40 minutes low-intensity walking on limited-carb days and 45 minutes circuit training on normal-carb days.

Week 2   2–5 cycle, Level B. Continue to exercise as in week 1.

Week 3   2–5 cycle, Level B. Increase intensity of circuit training by increasing weight.

Week 4   2–5 cycle, Level C. Continue to exercise as in week 3.

Week 5   2–5 cycle, Level C. Incorporate one day of slow-fast interval training on the elliptical machine on limited-carb days.

Week 6   2–5 cycle, Level C. Continue to exercise as in week 5.

After you've completed the initial six-week program, I recommend that women switch to a 1–3 regimen on Level B or C as a maintenance regimen.

Women

	MON	TUES	WED	THURS	FRI	SAT	SUN
EXERCISE	CIRCUIT TRAINING 60 MINUTES	ELLIPTICAL MACHINE SLOW/FAST 40 MINUTES	FAST WALK W/DUMBBELLS 60 MINUTES	ELLIPTICAL MACHINE 60 MINUTES	CIRCUIT TRAINING 60 MINUTES	OFF	OFF
DIET	NORMAL	LIMITED	LIMITED	LIMITED	NORMAL	LIMITED	LIMITED

Men may want to try increasing the number of normal-carb days in their regimen in order to gain muscle mass. I'll explain macrocycling regimens, in which the number of normal-carb days exceeds the number of limited-carb days, in more detail in Chapter 9, but in general, I recommend that men try a 7–7 regimen.

Tips for Exercisers

It takes time to build endurance and stamina. The mistake many people make is that they expect to see stamina improvement right away. When they don't drop weight or build muscle, they become disappointed and question the program's effectiveness. Or they drop the exercise program altogether.

In the beginning, don't make intensity your primary goal. Give your body time to adjust to the new routine. Here are your starting goals:

1. Set a routine for regular exercising. Try for at least a thirty minute period, three or four times a week.
2. Establish your number of miles run or walked each week.
3. Concentrate on the number of breaks you take during an exercise session. Keep the breaks short.

For example, let's say your goal per exercise session is three miles. Whether you feel energetic or not, no matter how many stops you make, you should try to complete your goal every time you exercise. I tell my clients, "No matter how you do it, you should cross that imaginary finish line. You can make 10 brief rest stops. You can walk and run. That's okay. What is important is to complete your daily, weekly, and monthly miles. It is important to stick to an exercise routine. That way, you're more likely to stay with it." Time yourself. Keep a personal record and try to improve it. Beating yourself can be a bigger thrill than watching a close baseball game.

I recommend walking and the elliptical machine for your aerobic workouts because they are both low impact on your ankle and knee joints. Running can put major stress on your ankles and knee joints, especially if you are severely overweight. Biking on a stationary bike, swimming, or running in the pool are also good aerobic options. In addition, you should focus on circuit training and do your walking with dumbbells. You can start running after you've achieved a healthy weight. If you wish to run, do it on the beach, on the dry sand. If you use a treadmill, run on a 2-to-4 percent incline. These options are more gentle to the joints.

Once damaged, joint cartilage does not normally regenerate completely. Accumulated over the time these chronic microinjuries eventually manifest as osteoarthritis, leading to restricted mobility, pain and disconfort later in your life. Prevention is key. Protect your joints now to avoid problems later in your life. The following measures may decrease your risk of joint degeneration:

1. Avoid running in the beginning of the program.
2. Concentrate on circuit training as a form of aerobic exercise instead of running or biking. The older you become the less running and more circuit training you should do.

3. Take joints support supplement regularly.
4. Avoid exercising when joints are sore.

In the early days, you will need a longer recovery period along with increased supplements to support your joints. I recommend formulas containing MSM, chondroitin sulfate, glucosamine, sea cucumber, Boswellia extract, gelatin, and hyaluronic acid for that time period to prevent joint damage. We'll discuss this in more detail in Chapter 10.

In addition, make sure you allow your body to recover after exercise. Muscle soreness is the body's normal reaction to physical stress. Muscle soreness tells you that the exercise was performed intensively and effectively. It means you can expect health and fat-loss benefits. Over time, as your fitness level improves, the episodes of soreness will lessen.

The rule of thumb: when you increase your physical activity, increase your nutritional support. Under physical stress, the body needs more vitamins, more minerals, more essential fatty acids and more amino acids. Make sure your food choices are nutritionally rich and include unrefined carbohydrates as a main energy source.

To accelerate recovery after exercise, consider taking or eating foods high in:
- Vitamin E (400 i.u.) at bedtime
- Coenzyme Q10, 120–1,000 mg
- Essential Fatty Acids, 5–15 g
- Vitamin C or Alpha Lipoic acid, 300 mg
- Lecithin 1,200 mg
- Calcium 1,200 mg

Again, we'll learn more about these in Chapter 10.

Doing Circuit Training Right

You'll begin circuit training right away in your exercise program. As we learned in Chapter 7, circuit training simply means that you are doing weight lifting or strength training exercises in a certain order, or circuit. The main thing is to start easy. Start by doing five repetitions at each station and work up to ten. Once you get comfortable with ten, up the ante to 15. When things begin to seem easy, test your new 1-RM lifting ability. If you could lift 100 pounds at the beginning, you will soon be able to lift 125 pounds, then 150. So increase the resistance of your lifts to 40 percent of your new 1-RM capability: 50 pounds instead of 40, etc.

If you are a beginner, start with a longer rest period—one to two minutes—between sets and reduce the rest interval as your fitness improves. Make sure that you exercise big muscles first such as leg muscles, buttocks, chest, and back. You can finish your circuit workout with a short, but intensive, run. Typically, 10 to 12 weight exercises are performed for the upper-body and 10 to 12 exercises for the lower-body. There are 15 repetitions of each exercise. As you raise your fitness level, allow no more than 30 seconds rest between each exercise. Keep your heart rate within your target zone, calculated as follows:

220 - age = Maximum Heart Rate (MHR)
upper limit of target heart rate: MHR × 0.9
lower limit of target heart rate = MHR × 0.6

You can purchase a heart rate monitor (from Nike, for example) and wear it during circuit training.

Circuit training may seem difficult for beginners since it requires a high level of fitness, but the benefits are outstanding. It improves muscular strength, cardiovascular system functioning and the general fitness level. People doing circuit training really feel alive.

Research shows that it increases lean body mass significantly. A three-pound gain in lean body mass can be expected with a corresponding decrease in relative fat mass.

There are many excellent books that describe weight training and circuit training, including *The Body Sculpting Bible* series by James Villepigue and Hugo Rivera, and you will want to either consult those or work with a personal trainer to be sure you learn the proper form for each exercise. But, to get you started, here is a basic circuit. You can vary the exact order, if necessary, but start with exercises that work larger muscles (for instance, chest and back) and then move on to exercises that work smaller muscles (biceps, triceps, and calves). Also, you'll see that there are a few aerobic exercises mixed into your circuit to keep your heart rate up.

Upper body weight lifting exercises:
Chest: Dumbbell Bench Press, Dumbbell Flyes, Push-Ups
Back: One-Arm Dumbbell Rows, Wide-Grip Pulldowns,
  Rowing on Machine (for 10 minutes)
Shoulders: Side Raises, Bent-Over Raises, Barbell Press
Biceps: Incline Dumbbell Curls, Seated Dumbbell Curls
Triceps: Dumbbell Extensions, Triceps Dips, Bench Dips

Lower body and ab exercises:
Abs: Floor Crunches, V-Ups
Quadriceps: Leg Extensions, Leg Press
Glutes: Dumbbell Squats, Treadmill Sprint (for 2 minutes) or
  Fast Biking (for 3 minutes)

DUMBBELL BENCH PRESS

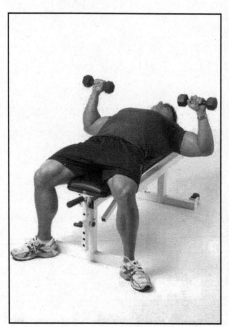 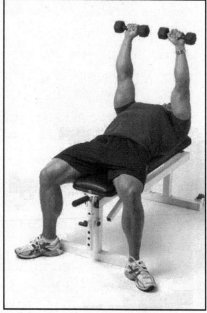

Lie back on a flat bench with your elbows out to the side and fore-arms perpendicular to the floor, grasping the dumbbells firmly with your palms facing forward. Press the weights up toward the ceiling. Return to your starting position, and repeat.

DUMBBELL FLYES

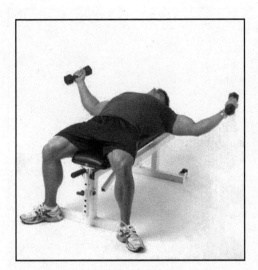 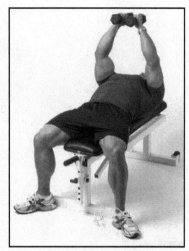

Lie back on a flat bench with your arms out to the side and elbows slightly bent, grasping the dumbbells firmly with your palms facing each other. Arc the weights towards each other, but keep your elbows bent, as if you are hugging a tree. Return to your starting position, and repeat.

PUSH-UPS

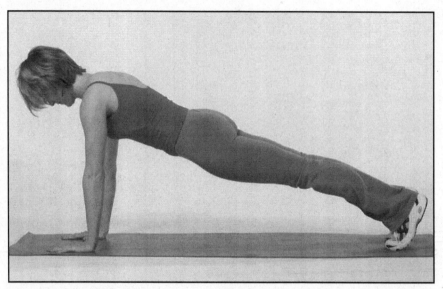

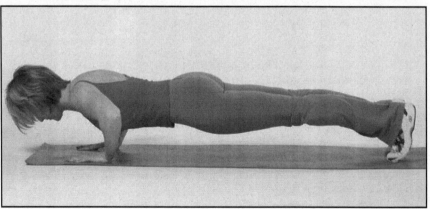

Prop yourself up on your hands and toes, facing down toward the floor with your arms straight. Lower yourself towards the floor, keeping your elbows out to the sides. Return to your starting position, and repeat.

ONE-ARM DUMBBELL ROWS

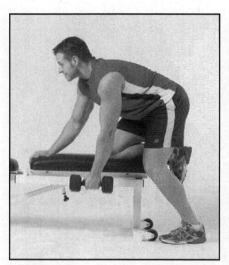 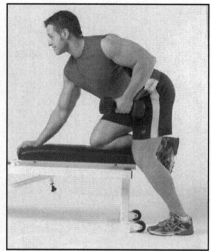

Kneel with your right knee and hand on a flat bench, holding a dumbbell in your left hand with your palm facing your body. Be sure to keep your back straight and parallel to the floor. Pull the weight up towards your left hip, as if you are trying to put it in your pocket, making sure your left elbow reaches the level of the torso. Return to your starting position, and repeat. Then switch sides.

WIDE-GRIP PULLDOWNS

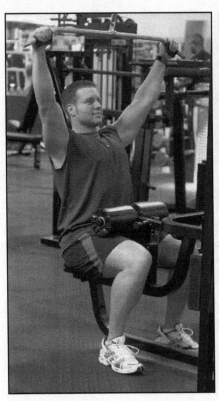 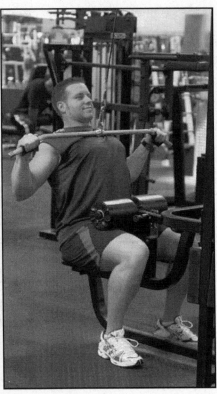

Sit at a pulldown machine with your feet flat on the floor and the thigh support snug. Keeping your hands more than shoulder-width apart, grasp the bar and pull down towards your chest. Return to your starting position, and repeat.

SIDE RAISES

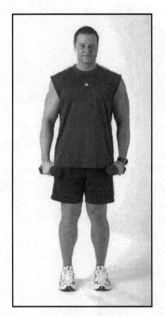 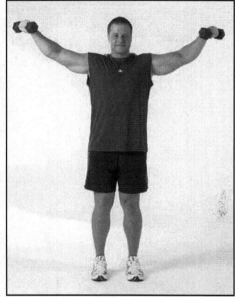

Stand with your feet hip-width apart, holding dumbbells with your palms facing each other. Raise your arms directly out to your sides until they reach shoulder level, keeping your elbows slightly bent. Return to your starting position, and repeat.

BENT-OVER RAISES

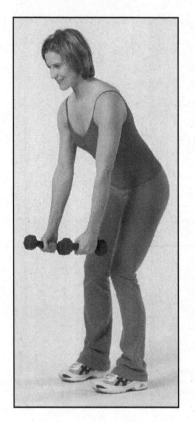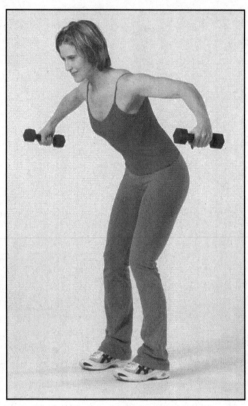

Start from the same position as the side raises, bend over at the hips, keeping your back straight and parallel to the floor, then raise your arms directly out to your sides until they reach shoulder level, keeping your elbows slightly bent. Return to your starting position, and repeat.

You can also do this exercise on a bench. Sit at an incline bench set at a 30-degree angle, facing the angled pad and holding dumbbells with your palms facing each other, then lift the dumbbells as described above.

BARBELL PRESS

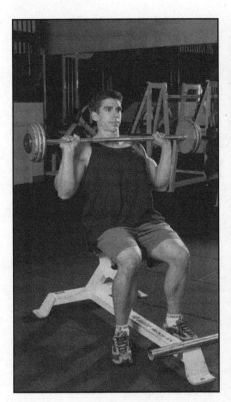 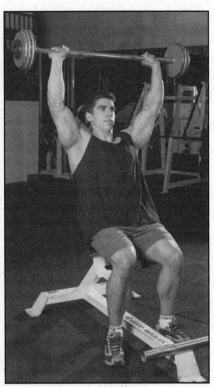

Sit at a bench with back support with your feet flat on the floor, holding a barbell across across your chest with your hands more than shoulder-width apart. Raise your arms directly overhead. Return to your starting position, and repeat.

INCLINE DUMBBELL CURL

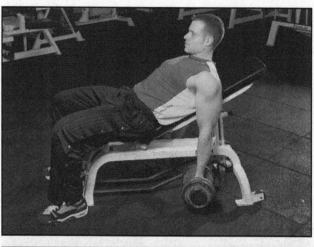

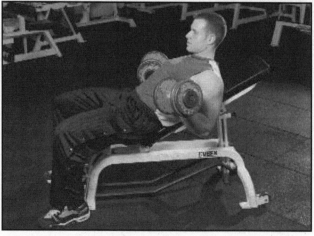

Sit at an incline bench set at a 45-degree angle, holding dumbbells with your palms facing up. Curl the weights up toward your shoulders, keeping your upper arm as still as possible. Return to your starting position, and repeat.

SEATED DUMBBELL CURL

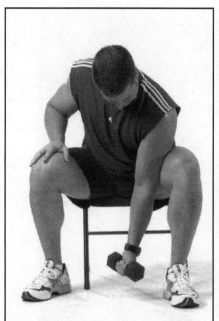 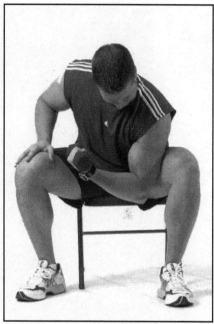

Sit at the edge of a chair or bench and bend over at the hips, sup-
porting your left arm on your left thigh. Hold a dumbbell in your
left hand and curl the weight up toward your shoulder, keeping
your upper arm as still as possible. Return to your starting position,
and repeat. Then switch sides.

DUMBBELL EXTENSIONS

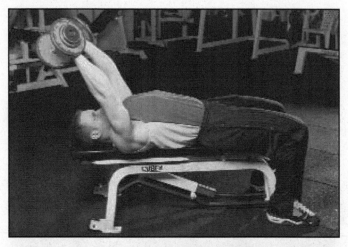

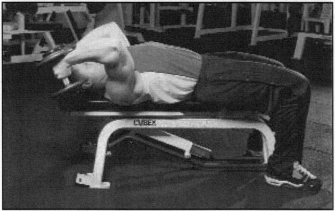

Lie back on a bench with your feet flat on the floor, holding dumbbells above your head with your arms extended. Lower the weights toward your head. Return to your starting position, and repeat.

TRICEPS DIPS

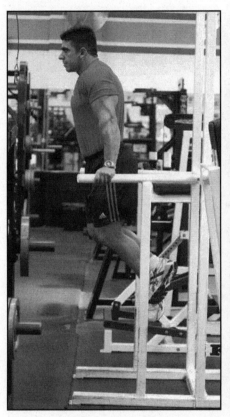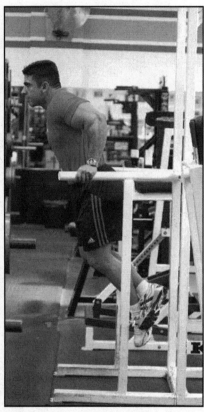

Place your hands on the parallel bars of a triceps dip machine, with your arms extended. Lower yourself toward the floor, keeping your elbows close your body. Return to your starting position, and repeat. If you need assistance, stand on the foot platform.

BENCH DIPS

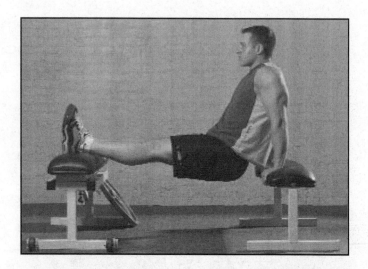

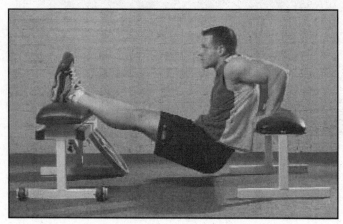

Place your feet on one bench and the palms of your hands on a second bench, facing forward and with your body suspended between the benches. Lower yourself toward the floor, keeping your elbows close to your body. Return to your starting positon, and repeat.

FLOOR CRUNCHES

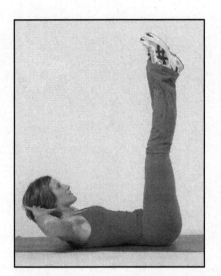 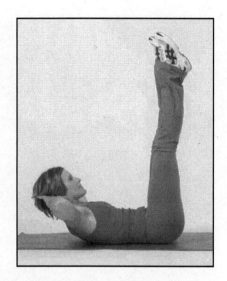

Lie on your back with your feet in the air and your hands by your neck. Curl your torso up toward your knees, focusing on tightening your abs as you do so. Return to your starting position, and repeat. If this is difficult, try it with your feet flat on the floor and knees bent.

V-Up

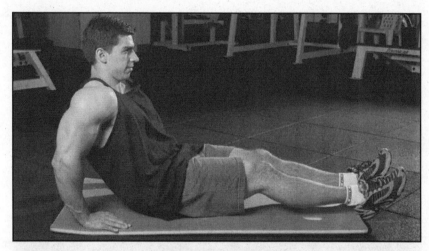

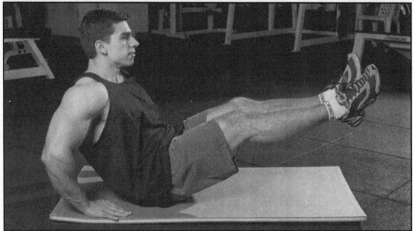

Sit on the floor with your arms slightly behind you and palms flat on the floor, leaning back to a 45-degree angle. Pull your knees towards your chest until your body makes a V, then push your legs straight out in front of you. Repeat this in-and-out motion without letting your legs touch the ground.

LEG EXTENSION

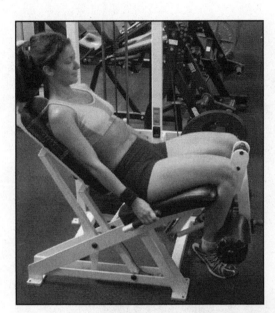

Sit at a leg extension machine with your back against the back pad, the back of your knees are pressed against the front of the seat, and your shins behind the roller pad. Extend your legs in front of you, lifting the roller pad. Return to your starting position, and repeat.

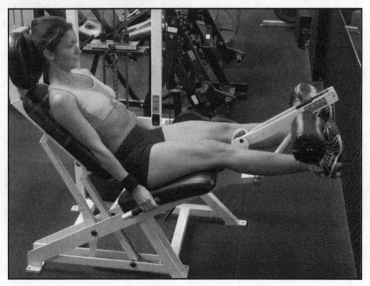

LEG PRESS

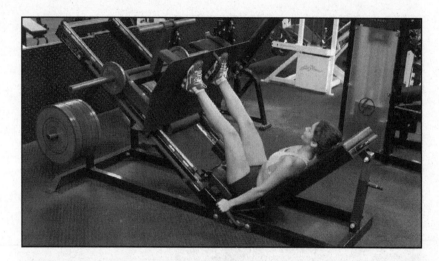

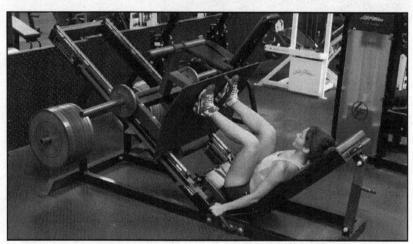

Sit at a leg press machine with your back against the back pad and feet flat against the plate. Extend your legs in front of you, pressing the platform away from you. Return to your starting position, and repeat.

DUMBBELL SQUAT

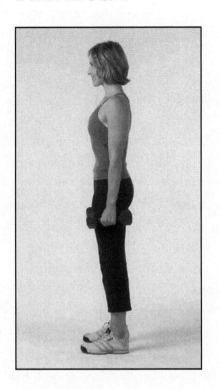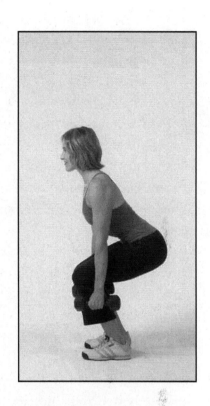

Stand with your feet hip-width apart, holding dumbbells with your palms facing each other. Lower yourself toward the floor, as if you were going to sit in an imaginary chair. Be sure to keep your knees in front of your toes. Return to your starting position, and repeat.

Doing Interval Training Right

Interval training can be done with any aerobic exercise. As we noted, I recommend the elliptical machine because it's easier on your joints. Start with small speed increments. For example, increase your speed a little for one minute. Then, slow down for a two-minute interval. This is known as Slow-Fast training.

While doing interval training, go faster than you usually do, but not too fast. Don't risk collapsing. Control your body movements all the time. It will be harder as you get more tired. Work yourself up to a pace where you can run for two minutes without stopping. Then rest for two to three minutes. As you improve, aim for shorter breaks.

Interval training has a number of variables that can be changed: the repetition time, the number of repetitions, and the rest interval time. The last one (rest interval time) is the most important. The amount of time your body rests defines how much lactic acid is removed from the muscles. The lactic acid is a byproduct of glycogen breakdown. The less you rest means more lactic acid remains in your muscles. In turn, a higher lactic acid level trains your body to operate better. Your muscles get used to it and this is exactly what you need. Keep your rest interval time fairly short, between 30 seconds and two minutes. Just make sure you perform at least six high-intensity repetitions per workout. Six to twelve repetitions are optimal. Following are a few examples of different intervals.

One-minute repetition with two-minute rests (about midway, there is one repetition at 95 percent of MAX effort). Start exercise session with 5 minutes of jogging. After the warm up accelerate to 85% of your maximum effort. Keep the speed for 1 minute. Slowdown to walking and rest while walking for 2 minutes. Repeat 12 times.

TIME	MAX EFFORT
5 minutes warm up	30 %
1 minutes	85 %
2 minutes	WALKING
1 minutes	85 %
2 minutes	WALKING
30 seconds	95 %
2 minutes	WALKING
1 minutes	85 %
2 minutes	WALKING
1 minutes	85 %
2 minutes	WALKING
1 minutes	65 %
2 minutes	WALKING

TOTAL: 23 MINUTES

30-second repetitions with 1-minute rests (about midway, there is one repetition at 95 percent of MAX effort). The running speed is faster than in previous example.

TIME	MAX EFFORT
5 minutes warm up	30 %
30 seconds	90 %
1 minute	WALKING
30 seconds	90 %
1 minute	WALKING
30 seconds	95 %
1 minute	WALKING
30 seconds	90 %
1 minute	WALKING
30 seconds	90 %
1 minute	WALKING
30 seconds	90 %
1 minute	WALKING

TOTAL: 14 MINUTES

Slow-Fast training. Here your "rest" intervals are faster than a walk but your "run" intervals are slower than in previous examples, so your overall effort remains relatively high.

TIME	MAX EFFORT
5 minutes warm up	30 %
2 minutes	65 %
4 minutes	30 %
2 minutes	65 %
4 minutes	30 %
2 minutes	65 %
4 minutes	30 %
2 minutes	65 %
4 minutes	30 %
2 minutes	65 %
4 minutes	30 %
2 minutes	65 %
4 minutes	30 %

TOTAL: 41 MINUTES

Breaking the Plateau

As you have come to know, the body is highly adaptive. There is both good and bad news in that statement. The good news is that your body will adapt to a new eating pattern—fewer refined carbohydrates—which leads to a decrease of appetite and cravings. The bad news is the body will adapt to decreased calorie intake by decreasing its BMR. In short, your body goes into an efficiency mode and learns to live on fewer calories. The human body always finds a way to operate in an energy-efficient way. Evolution made us highly focused on survival. The previous events of food shortage, when humans did not have abundance of food, taught our bodies to find the most efficient ways to survive, that is, to live longer on less energy intake. Severe calorie shortage, such as less than 1,200 calories, turns on such mechanisms; the body adjusts to the extremes by slowing down the metabolism and fat loss slows down as well.

The fat-loss process is not linear. Rather it is like a garden-path stairway with long, flat flagstone steps. Many times you may spend a long time on one step and seemingly will not move any further. Sometimes it takes a lot of effort to make just one step. If that happens, consider these suggestions:

- Review your diet and make adjustments. For example, use Stevia Plus instead of Splenda. Stevia is a natural herb while Splenda is not. Decrease the fat in your diet — fat has more than twice the calories of protein or carbohydrates. Finally, increase your use of whey protein, egg whites, and L-Carnitine.
- Review your exercises. Change them and if possible, change the times when you exercise. Another way to change your schedule is to split your exercises into two sessions. On weekends, adopt morning (before breakfast) and evening sessions. Incorporate one interval (stop-and-go sprint) training session each week. Weight lifting? Change the number of repetitions. Pick up heavier weights and start doing 4–8 reps if you were doing 8-12 reps. Change the rest period from 1–2 minutes to 2–3 minutes or vise versa. Start circuit training with minimum rest between exercises. Mix the intensities. For example, one day do 20 minutes of interval training, another day bike for 60 minutes using the highest resistance level but at low speed. Do anything you can think of to keep your exercise routine, from your body's perspective, unpredictable.
- Extend the number of limited-carb days in your regimen.
- Finally, take a week or two off from exercising. An overtired body resists any weight loss attempts.

A Special Exercise—Increase Your Metabolism

You have learned that to increase metabolism, you need to make sure that you consume your daily calorie needs. But you can do more. Besides consuming enough calories, you can perform anabolic hormone releasing exercises (MAX Effort exercises). It takes only 15 minutes a day, but is the most effective way to boost HGH and testosterone production. Dozens of studies have shown that a burst of power during heavy weight lifting leads to an increase in blood HGH and testosterone concentration.

Caution: this type of exercise is not for everyone. Only absolutely healthy individuals who have previous experience with heavy weight lifting should be doing it. If you are not accustomed with heavy weight lifting, start with moderate weight and progress gradually over a period of 12 to 24 months. Recent studies also show that a burst of heavy exercise performed by untrained individuals can invoke heart attack, blood vessels rupture, stroke or even eye damage! So be cautious!

The MAX Effort exercise can be done as a bench press or a leg press. It can also be performed as a deadlift or barbell squat, but only by experienced weight lifters since if done incorrectly, it may cause severe injuries. Before starting this exercises review machine instructions and consult a personal trainer for proper technique. For example, it is very important to have a correct starting position (90 degree leg bent) when perform leg press and perform all movements slowly.

How to perform the MAX Effort bench press:

Use the Smith machine. It has safety hooks that eliminate the need for a spotter. The Nautilus press machine can be used also.

Caution: Do not perform this exercise with a free bar without a spotter! Always warm up with a few sets using medium weight.

1. Find your 1-RM (1-Repetition Maximum).

2. Deduct 30 pounds from 1-RM weight.

3. Do 8 sets of 3 repetitions. Women can do 6 sets of 3 repetitions each. ·

That's it. You're done. It should take you only 15 minutes to complete this exercise. You have to force yourself to leave the gym. Do not proceed with any additional exercises on this day except stretching.

Stay with 3 reps for a while (a month or two) before moving to 2 reps and increasing the weight. I do not recommend 1 rep since it may cause injuries. Check your 1-RM once a week.

This type of exercise is meant to increase anabolic hormone release. If performed properly, without any additional exercises, it provides significant anti-aging benefits. You will start feeling more energetic, especially at the end of the day. The effect may last for up to two days. If you do not feel increase in energy level then review your exercise program. You may be doing too much exercising with little amount of rest that restrains the anabolic hormones release.

Make the day when you perform anabolic hormones releasing exercise (MAX Effort) your easy training day. Why are any additional exercises not recommended on this day? It may reverse anabolism into catabolism, the opposite of what we are looking for. Exercise, if performed intensively, leads to a post-exercise catabolic state. Cortisol is released as a result of the physical stress. This is one of the reasons why I recommend consuming carbohydrate-heavy meals right after weight lifting session—to stop cortisol release and prevent catabolism.

The CARB CYCLING DIET

9

Microcycling and Macrocycling

The Carb Cycling Diet regimens described so far have mostly been examples of microcycling. Any regimen with one normal-carb day at a time in the cycle (1–2, 1–3, 1–4,1–5, 1–6) promotes fat loss and are considered microcycling. These regimens are designed primarily for women and for those who do not exercise.

When the number of normal-carb days exceeds one (for instance, 2–2, 2–4, 3–3, and so on), the regimen becomes a macrocycling. Macrocycling is used to build muscle. In the men's programs we've presented so far, we have kept the number of normal-carb days low (equal to, or below, the number of limited-carb days) in order to initiate fat loss in the first six weeks. In order to build muscles, the number of normal-carb days needs to be increased. With macrocycling, you have to build muscles first, and then you can focus on losing extra fat that might have accumulated during the muscle-building phase.

Professional bodybuilders take this philosophy to the extreme. They use bulking and cutting cycles that may last for a few weeks at a time. During the bulking phase they lift heavy weights and consume a lot of calories. Some fat is usually accumulated during this phase. Then they switch to cutting phase when they drop their calorie intake by restricting carbohydrates and fat and perform a lot of aerobic exercise.

While the bodybuilder's routine is extreme, you can use these same principles if at any time you detect that your muscles are becoming weak and you need to give your body a better nutritional jolt. Switch to macrocycling. In fact, any time you feel you need a break from dieting (which I recommend that you do regularly in order to increase your metabolism), switch to macrocycling and try to build some muscles. Don't worry that you'll build too much. Muscles are much easier to lose than to build!

The more normal carb days in your regimen the better for building muscles. That is because muscles need some time to grow; they do not grow on the same day you exercise them but rather on the following days. For this reason, you will want to rest from exercise on some normal-carb days during your macrocycling regimen.

Here is an example of a 5-4 regimen:

SUN	MON	TUES	WED	THURS	FRI	SAT	SUN	MON
STRENGTH TRAINING UPPER BODY	STRENGTH TRAINING LOWER BODY	OFF	STRENGTH TRAINING UPPER BODY	STRENGTH TRAINING LOWER BODY	OFF	AEROBIC EXERCISE RUNNING	AEROBIC EXERCISE CIRCUIT TRAINING	AEROBIC EXERCISE ELLIPTICAL MACHINE
NORMAL	NORMAL	NORMAL	NORMAL	NORMAL	LIMITED	LIMITED	LIMITED	LIMITED

Again, women probably will want to maintain a lower number of normal-carb days even in a macrocycling regimen: I recommend that women start with a 2–5 regimen when they first begin macrocycling. Men can try a 7–7 regimen. You can increase the number of normal carb days to make sure that you exercise the same muscle at least twice before starting limited-carb days. On normal-carb days, make sure that you consume about 300 calories more than your body needs. For truly serious fitness enthusiasts, working up to a rigorous 21–7 regimen will deliver better muscle-building results.

Here is an example of a 2-5 regimen:

	MON	TUES	WED	THURS	FRI	SAT	SUN
EXERCISE	OFF	ELLIPTICAL MACHINE	CIRCUIT TRAINING	OFF	RUNNING	STRENGTH TRAINING	STRENGTH TRAINING
DIET	LIMITED	LIMITED	LIMITED	LIMITED	LIMITED	NORMAL	NORMAL

During the normal-carb days, do weight lifting only—no aerobic exercises like running, swimming or even circuit training. While doing weight lifting focus on the selected muscle and exercise it until its failure before moving to another muscle. During the following protein-packed, limited-carb days, do circuit training and those aerobic cardio-vascular, running and biking exercises, which aim at conditioning the heart and lungs.

Supplement these exercises with calcium at a rate of 1,000 to 1,750 mg a day. Calcium plays a major role in muscle contraction. When released from its storage, it causes the muscles to contract. If you don't supplement your daily intake with calcium, the body might rob it from your teeth and bones.

Here are some other tips that will help you build muscles:

1. Progress in weights. Pick up heavier weights. While untrained individuals show a great progress in the beginning of any exercise program the progression slows down after the initial phase. To continue progression the heavier weights need to be used—60 percent and more of 1-RM.

   General rule: Pick up a weight that allows you to do no more than 8 repetitions. Once you can complete 12 repetitions with that weight, increase it so you will be forced to go back to 8 repetitions.

2. Exercise regularly. The muscle size and strength diminish if the load is not applied regularly. The best time interval for exercising the same muscle is 2 times per week.

3. Achieve muscle failure. In order to achieve the tear of muscle myofibrils the last 2 sets need to be finished with muscle failure, no matter how many repetitions it takes. It is important to work out the muscles really hard, to actually damage them on the cellular level (to cause a microtrauma to the myofibrils), so that new muscle myofibrils can grow. For this reason you need to concentrate on one muscle in a time and make sure you put enough hard stress on it by exercising it to the point of failure. Most people merely exercise—making their muscles move, not going out of their "comfort zone"—which is not enough to build muscle.

Carb Cycling Diet and Exercise at a Glance

If your goal is to lose fat, use microcycling regimens.

If your goal is to build muscles, use macrocycling regimens.

Perform strength training exercises on normal-carb days.

Perform aerobic (cardio) exercises on limited-carb days.

Eat refined carbs only after strength training exercise.

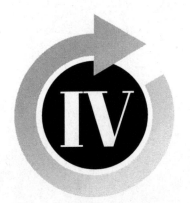

Maintenance and Adaptation

10

The World of Sports Supplements

Many useful supplements are advertised today, but if you are tempted to use all of them, don't. Your body won't be able to handle the load. You need to concentrate on ones that are safe and have multiple health-promoting benefits. These supplements will be described in this chapter.

The claims made by supplement distributors often are not proven. One such dubious case deals with substances that claim to stimulate the pituitary gland to produce Human Growth Hormone. The public may be misled by the anti-aging benefits the advertiser boasts about. Usually the distributor fails to mention that these benefits were registered only after the Human Growth Hormone was given by injection in high dosages. The list of ineffective and useless supplements could fill a very big book, so let's concentrate on some useful ones.

Some of these supplements, most notably hormones, should only be taken under the strict supervision of a physician. Before you take any supplements, though, you should consult with your doctor to make sure they are safe and will not interact with any medications you may be taking. Remember, most supplements are not regulated by the federal government so you will need to do your own research to determine if they are safe and effective.

Metabolism Boosters

If metabolism slows down over time through the decrease of hormones, it would seem to make sense that taking hormones would combat aging. This, at least, is the premise behind hormone replacement therapies including HGH, DHEA, and sex hormones. These all require a doctor's supervision. As I mentioned earlier, because of its high cost it is not suitable for everyone, and it may have adverse side effects. Boosting your metabolism through the Carb Cycling Diet and Exercise Plan is much safer and cheaper.

It is difficult to find a supplement that will raise the basal metabolic rate although many product labels claim that they increase metabolism. The basal metabolic rate directly correlates with your age and is affected by the levels of Human Growth Hormone, sex hormones, DHEA, and thyroid hormones in your blood. The older you get, the lower the hormone level, and the slower your basal metabolic rate. Here's what we do know about hormones.

HUMAN GROWTH HORMONE (HGH)

HGH is a hormone—nature's own stimulant—that you can use to fight fat. It gets to the root of the problem by increasing the basal metabolic rate and provides anti-aging benefits as well.

The HGH molecule is large, like insulin, which means it cannot be absorbed through human membranes. So Human Growth Hormone is taken as injections. The injections are effective but expensive, starting at $300 a month. However, be cautious. As of today, there are no long-term studies showing safety of HGH supplementation.

There is a good side to the story. MAX Effort exercise is the natural way to increase Human Growth Hormone. Studies show that the more intense the exercise, the more HGH and other anabolic hormones are released. The more often Max Effort exercise you perform, the more often HGH and testosterone will be released into your blood naturally. Elderly people also show increased levels of these hormones after intense exercise. As a result, most of them who exercise with heavy weights don't really need Viagra or Cialis.

HGH SECRETAGOGES

Secretagoges are substances meant to stimulate internal gland functions, such as that involved in releasing Human Growth Hormone. Many commercial products sold in health food stores and on the Internet claim they can increase your Human Growth Hormone level by up to 400 percent. In truth, they cannot. Though some people report sleep improvement and other favorable effects after using these products, these results are attributed to the relaxing action of L-arginine on blood vessels. L-arginine, an amino-acid, is usually a part of the blend.

Experiments show that some amino acids increase Human Growth Hormone levels in the blood if taken as injections in large doses over a short period of time. The effects are not the same if taking orally and in long term usage.

The effects of orally administered drugs are different from intravenous or intramuscular injection. To achieve an effective level in the blood, the oral dosage should be two to three times higher than the intravenous dosage. That's because oral doses undergo liver detoxification before reaching the tissues. One publication reported that high intravenous doses of L-arginine (4 g) stimulated Human Growth Hormone secretion in young athletes. (This effect was not noticed in older people.) By then, the secretagoge boom already had gotten started. To achieve this useful concentration (4 grams of L-arginine in the blood), a person would have to take 12 grams of Arginine powder (that's 24 capsules of 500 mg each). Unfortunately, over time the stimulating action tends to subside because the body adjusts to the stimulation. The bottom line is that the Human Growth Hormone secretagoges available on today's market are not practical. Scientists are currently working on a new generation of secretagoges that will be more effective than those currently available.

DHEA

The DHEA hormone is produced by the adrenal glands. It is the precursor—or granddaddy—of all sex hormones. As we age, the secretion of DHEA declines leading to a decline of sex hormone production. Supplementing DHEA would seem to be an effective way to restore the level of sex hormones, but I don't recommend the use of DHEA without doctor's supervision. As we age more and more, testosterone gets converted into estrogen naturally. Any extra amounts of testosterone will quickly transform into estrogen. Thus increases estrogen in unhealthy proportion with testosterone. When natural balance of hormones is shifted it may lead to prostate cancer and gynecomastia, which translates as breast gland enlargement in men. In women it can increase the risk of estrogen-related cancers.

7-KETO

Fortunately, there is a safe alternative to DHEA: 7-Keto. It is a byproduct of DHEA conversion. It does not convert into sex hormones, but it does effectively increase metabolism, the condition you seek. Studies report that its use leads to fat loss accompanied by an increase in both energy and metabolism. Even at high dosages, there are no negative side effects reported. I recommend one 100-

mg tablet after breakfast or one hour before exercise taken in 1 month courses.

MELATONIN

Melatonin is a hormone produced in the brain during sleep. Its production increases during sleep and lowers during a daytime thus regulating body's day and night cycles. It helps the body to get rest and recover form the stress. I recommend taking it periodically when you feel tired or exhausted from exercise but no more than once a week since every day usage may diminish anabolic hormones secretion. Take 1 capsule (3 mg) once a week.

THYROID HORMONE

The thyroid hormone has a fat loss effect but also has dangerous long-term consequences. If you take a thyroid hormone, your body's thyroid stimulating hormone will be suppressed and take a long time to return to normal. Only those who are suffering from hypothyroidism and under a physician's supervision should use this hormone. Otherwise, avoid thyroid hormone! Make sure that supplements you take do not contain even small quantities of thyroid hormones.

L-TYROSINE FOR THYROID DEFICIENCY

L-Tyrosine is a key amino acid in thyroid hormone synthesis. It is a precursor of thyroxine, a thyroid hormone, as well as the neurotransmitters adrenaline and noradrenaline. Patients with a thyroxine deficiency experience excess weight gain, depression, cold hands and feet, difficulty concentrating, and a decreased basal metabolic rate. L-Tyrosine supplementation might restore the thyroxine level to normal. The recommended daily dosage is 500 mg.

Note: If you have elevated blood pressure or any heart conditions do not use L–Tyrosine.

Kelp for Iodine

Kelp is a source of natural iodine. Combined with L–Tyrosine it forms a thyroid hormone. To support normal functioning of thyroid gland, take two capsules of kelp with one capsule of L–Tyrosine (500 mg) every other day in the morning. Do not exceed the recommended dosage of kelp because heart palpitations and sleep disturbance may result. If you are a sushi lover, remember that the dark green nori (laver) that sushi comes wrapped in is pure kelp.

Energy-Increasing Supplements
Caffeine

Caffeine, a well-known stimulant, has been proven to be safe even in high doses. Professional athletes use it before their workout sessions to increase exercise performance and bring workout intensity to the highest possible level.

Many people are often advised to abstain from consuming caffeinated beverages. But in the case of those who exercise, the studies indicate that caffeine stimulates exercise performance with a mild diuretic effect. There was no evidence of fluid-electrolyte imbalances or any other health hazard.

A daily intake of caffeine equal to five cups of coffee at one sitting (about 500 mg of caffeine) has no side effects. With regular consumption of caffeine, a person may develop a tolerance to many of its effects.

Guarana seeds

Guarana is an herb native to the Amazon region. The guarana seeds contain caffeine that combined with tannins, starch, and resinous substances that allow caffeine to absorb slowly thus providing all day long energy support. Take one capsule in the morning and one at lunchtime.

DMAE

Dimethylaminoethanol (DMAE) is another safe and effective supplement that increases energy levels. DMAE is a natural substance produced in the brain. It is involved in the synthesis of acetylcholine. It also improves mental functioning. Take one capsule in the morning together with two capsules of kelp and one of L-Tyrosine. Add Vitamin B-complex (B-50). These vitamins are important for improved energy production.

Note: If you have elevated blood pressure or any heart conditions do not use DMAE.

COENZYME Q-10

Coenzyme Q-10 is essential for the production of the high-energy phosphate, adenosine triphosphate (ATP). Coenzyme Q-10 is an excellent antioxidant, which means it will bond with the free radical molecules formed because of increased oxygen turnover during aerobic exercises. Free radicals are molecules responsible for developing more than 80 diseases, including heart disease, cancer, arthritis and the degenerative conditions of aging. The effective daily dose for coenzyme Q-10 is above 120 mg. This ability to deliver both increased endurance and protection from free radicals makes it the best supplement to take when doing aerobic exercise.

NADH (NICOTINAMIDE ADENINE DINUCLEOTIDE)

NADH is the principal carrier of electrons in the oxidation of molecules that produce energy in the body's cells. It is the body's most powerful antioxidant and is 300 times more powerful than Vitamin E or C. Like Q-10, it increases energy levels and provides protection from free radicals, making it another excellent supplement to take when doing aerobic exercise.

Diet Pills

Everyone who is trying to lose weight faces the question, "Are those pills really effective and should I use them or not?" These kinds of supplements (Thermo Gain, Hydroxycut, Xenadrine, etc.) suppress appetite and increase energy level. When used alone they can be considered as a temporary solution to permanent problem. I advise my patients to rely on these pills only in following scenarios:

1. In the beginning of a diet program, when your behavior is changing, but insulin secretion has not yet adjusted to the smaller amounts of food you eat.
2. Occasional, short-term use when breaking through a plateau.
3. Short-term usage as stimulants before a workout.

How to Use Supplements

Here is a list that you may consult when you go shopping for vitamins, minerals, and sports food supplements for the Carb Cycling Diet. They are available at most health food stores.

TAKE ANYTIME AS A SNACK

- Whey protein. Use it as a shake or add it to your favorite nonfat yogurt.
- Branched Chain Amino Acids (BCAA), three 1,000 mg capsules. Carry some with you on the go.

TO HELP KEEP BLOOD SUGAR STEADY

Any weight loss supplement that contains chromium and vanadium.

WHEN YOU FEEL A CRAVING FOR SWEETS

- Alpha Lipoic Acid, 300 mg.
- L-Carnitine Liquid, to prevent cravings for sweets and food. A small bottle is convenient to carry when you are on the go. The brand I recommend is CarniTech Liquid Carnitine Complex made by Universal Nutrition.
- Ultra Sugar Control (Made by Nature's Plus) or Ultimate Carb Phaser 1000 (Made by Biochem).

FOR ENERGY

- DMEA, 250, mg.
- Vitamin B-50. Made by Now Foods.
- Japanese green tea (sencha tea). Made by YamamotoYama. Can be ordered on Internet.

Note: If you have high blood pressure, do not use DMEA and L-Tyrosine.

PRE-EXERCISE MORNING SUPPLEMENTS

- 7-Keto. One 100-mg tablet an hour before exercise or after breakfast.
- DMEA, kelp, and L-Tyrosine. In the morning, take one capsule of DMAE together with two capsules of kelp and one of L-Tyrosine.
- Vitamin B-Complex. These vitamins are important for improved energy production.
- Coenzyme Q-10, 120 mg. for beginners to 1,000 mg. for hard-working advanced exercisers. This is the best supplement to take before doing aerobic exercises. It is a powerful anti-oxidant to defend your body against oxygen radicals when doing aerobics.

- NADH, which comes in tiny pill form, is 300 times more powerful than Vitamin C or E in fighting radicals. A good supplement to take before doing aerobic exercises.
- Extreme Energy Shot, from Arizona Beverage Co. If you cannot find this product, which seems to be not widely available, try to find an energy sports drink that contains both fructose and caffeine.

Note: If you have high blood pressure, do not use DMEA and L-Tyrosine.

POST-EXERCISE SUPPLEMENTS
- Whey Protein

FOR JOINT RECOVERY AFTER EXERCISE
- Vitamin E, 400 i.u. at bedtime.
- Vitamin C, 1,000 mg.
- Alpha Lipoic acid, 300 mg.
- Lecithin softgels, 1,200 mg.
- Calcium. 1,000 to 1,750 mg. (1,200 is the RDA for seniors.)
- Joint support formulas.
- Gelatin. NutraJoint. Made by Knox.

FOR LIMITED-CARB DAYS
- Kelp capsules, one or two only.
- Omega-3, Omega-6, Omega-9 oils. On limited-carb (high protein) days, take 5–15 grams a day.

IF YOU ARE OVERWEIGHT OR OBESE

To protect joints the joint support formulas are recommended for overweight people. These formulas should include:

- Glucosamine
- Chondroitin sulfate
- MSM
- Sea cucumber
- Boswellia extract
- Hyaluronic acid

You will find more information about where to find supplements in the Resource section. Please remember to consult your physician before you start any supplements.

The CARB CYCLING DIET

11

Maintaining the Program/Common Questions and Answers

Be realistic. Don't expect to see changes overnight. It took you years to get into your present condition. It takes time to recover. Be persistent and disciplined. After a few weeks of practicing carbohydrate cycling, your body will adjust by lowering the insulin secretion. How will you know that it has happened? Your cravings for refined carbohydrates will subside. You will realize that you do not need sweet desserts or ice cream anymore. You will not be hungry as often, and you will start to eat smaller amounts of food. Along with these changes, your weight undoubtedly will go down.

If you start with Program 2, remember that the introductory 1–1 (for women) or 2–2 (for men) regimens are merely the gateway to the Carb Cycling Diet. Do not expect a fat loss while you are on this preliminary regimen.

The Carb Cycling Exam

Now is the time for your final test. Let's assume someone important has planned a big family dinner for 4 p.m. on Sunday. Which of the answers below would be the best choice of action to prevent fat deposition?

    A. Run slowly for 30 minutes at 8 p.m. (A slow aerobic run burns more fat.)

    B. Run for 20 minutes doing 10 sprints at 3 p.m. (to increase hunger).

    C. Don't eat high-fat food at dinner.

    D. Don't eat refined carbohydrates at dinner.

While all answers A to D look like wise actions to take, by now you should be able to pick Choice B as the most effective of the lot. By the way, many well-educated personal trainers and even PhDs in nutrition fail this test. When it comes to party time, not many of us want to be observers or selective food eaters.

Common Questions and Answers about the Carb Cycling Diet

DIET

    Q. When is the best time to eat refined carbohydrates?

    A. During the first two hours after you exercise. If you are not exercising, for breakfast.

Q. Do normal-carb days cause difficulties in controlling blood sugar?

A. No. On the first limited-carb day, your insulin level quickly returns to a low value.

Q. Can I mix Level B and Level C restriction during the week?

A. Yes, you can. For example:

	MON	TUES	WED	THURS	FRI	SAT	SUN
EXERCISE	STRENGTH TRAINING	RUNNING	OFF	EM	STRENGTH TRAINING	OFF	OFF
DIET	NORMAL	LIMITED	LIMITED	LIMITED	NORMAL	LIMITED	LIMITED
LEVEL		B	C	B		C	C

Q. How do you monitor progress?

A. Weigh yourself every morning. One or two pounds of weight gain after a normal carb day may be attributed to food and water retention. Three pounds of gain should alert you to take action.

Q. I need to lose fat fast. Can I lower my daily calorie intake below Weight × 8 number?

A. There are no quick fixes for fat loss. Time and persistence is a key. If you go below this number you would lose large amount of muscle that is much easier to lose than to build. Instead, take healthier approach—refrain eating refined carbs on normal-carb days and stay above your Weight × 8 cal number on limited-carb days.

Q. Can I increase the number of limited-carb days beyond seven?

A. Occasionally you can. Generally, I do not recommend this since it slows down the metabolism.

Q. Can I eat white rice on Level B?

A. Yes, you can in small quantities, but brown and wild rice are preferred choices.

Q. How can I switch to the Carb Cycling Diet if I am currently on another diet?

A. If you are on a calorie-restricted diet (Atkins, South Beach or other) women who exercise should start with a 1–3 regimen. Men who exercise can start with a 7–7 regimen. Those who do not exercise should start on a 1–6 regimen.

Q. What can I eat to satisfy cravings for sweets after aerobic exercise? I often feel cravings for sweets right after walking.

A. Fruit is a good choice, for example bananas or apples. Remember, fruit is allowed on limited-carb days. Another good choice is a whey protein mix with nonfat yogurt.

EXERCISE

Q. When is the best time to exercise to burn more fat?

A. Early in the morning, before breakfast. Low intensity exercise on an empty stomach will burn large amount of fat.

Q. What do I do, if I skip exercise?

A. Make that day a Level C day with very limited carbs.

Q. How do you control your breathing while exercising?

A. Most runners breathe in a 2:2 ratio rhythmic to their steps. They take two steps as they inhale; and two more steps as they exhale. But when running slowly, they often breathe in a 3:3 ratio.

Q. Are breaks okay while exercising?

A. Running: Breaks during your run are okay if your break time does not exceed two minutes.

Weight Lifting: Breaks between sets and exercises during weight lifting should be between 1 and 3 minutes.

Q. What is 85 percent of MAX Effort?

A. 100 percent is your maximum effort. For example, it is the maximum speed that you can run a 100-meter sprint. In weight lifting it is the maximum weight that you can push.

Q. Can I use other exercises on limited-carb days?

A. Yes, you can. It does not matter what aerobic exercise you do. In the gym you can move from one machine to another. One of the reasons I recommend alternating aerobic exercises is to prevent adaptation; the body adjusts to the same exercise. If you cannot run or you are a beginner, walk with dumbbells. Women can use three-pound dumbbells. Men can use three- to eight-pound dumbbells. If you are a beginner, start with three-pound weights and work up. Carrying those weights does make a difference. Lift the weights over your head. Hold them out in front of you, at arms' length. Swing them back and forth. Do anything to give your arms, chest and shoulder muscles a mild workout.

Indoor activities: Dumbbells can be used for a stair-master or for walking on a treadmill on an incline.

Outdoor activities: Dumbbells can be utilized while walking. Hold a comfortable weight dumbbell in each hand, flex and extend your arms with each step. The park benches are great exercise tools as well. They are at a comfortable knee height and may be used for step aerobic exercises.

METABOLISM AND AGING

Q. Should I create a Positive Calorie Balance in order to increase metabolism?

A. The Positive Calorie Balance (approximately 300 calories more than Daily Calorie Needs) is desirable for those who concentrate on muscle building. If you are not, you can stay within Daily Calorie Needs.

Q. Why don't we lose fat as we age?

A. While the secretion of most anabolic hormones decline, one anabolic hormone secretion increase—insulin. This hormone is mainly responsible for depositing fat. The body is unable to use fat for energy when insulin blood concentration is high.

ADAPTING THE CARB CYCLING DIET

Q. I tried the Carb Cycling Diet for 6 months but could not resist refined carb cravings on limited-carb days. Is anything else I can try?

A. As a last resort, you can adjust the Carb Cycling Diet to cycle calories without restricting refined carb intake. You won't get all of the health benefits of the full Carb Cycling Diet, but you will at least be able to get to a healthy weight.

This form of calorie cycling is suitable for those who have a hard time restricting their refined carbohydrate intake. Try cycling calories without restricting refined carbs. Follow the same cycling regimens described in this book but instead of restricting carbs on your limited days, focus on calories. So, there are no restrictions in food choices, only the amount of consumed food is important.

On calorie-restricted days you eat less than your Daily Calorie Needs. You still can eat your favorite refined carbs, such as white bread or even ice cream, just in small quantities. On normal-calorie days, you should consume your Daily Calorie Needs or a little bit more.

For those who exercise, follow this simple guideline: Eat less food and do aerobic exercise on calorie-restricted days. Eat more food and do intensive (anaerobic) strength training on normal-calorie days. That is the least restrictive diet regimen ever developed! You do not have to sacrifice food you love. You just need to adjust exercise to the amount of food you eat. The calorie cycling concept makes the life of a carb cycling dieter easier as well. If you occasionally fail your limited-carb day by eating a Snickers bar, for example, do not panic.

Q. I am on 1–3 regimen but have a hard time keeping track of normal-carb days.

A. You can combine 1–3 regimen with 1–2. In this case you can have your normal carb day on the same day during the week—Sunday and Thursday. You want to go a little bit deeper into carb restriction (Level C) on Friday and Saturday. Here is an example of one week:

	SUN	MON	TUES	WED	THURS	FRI	SAT	SUN
EXERCISE	CIRCUIT TRAINING	OFF	RUN LOW	EM LOW	CIRCUIT TRAINING	OFF	HIIT HIGH	CIRCUIT TRAINING
DIET	NORMAL	LIMITED	LIMITED	LIMITED	NORMAL	LIMITED	LIMITED	NORMAL
LEVEL		B	B	B		C	C	

The CARB CYCLING DIET

A Parting Word

The Carb Cycling Diet gives you the luxury of eating forbidden foods. In return you need to make an effort to eat it at the right times. Is it difficult? Think about people on the Atkins diet. They are denied French fries and mom's cake—for the rest of their lives.

Be disciplined, but give yourself time and learn from your mistakes. If you do not see results within four weeks, don't be disappointed. Learn—and learn to adjust. And remember that exercise makes a huge difference. Even a short time spent exercising is better then none.

If you can't spend one hour a day to exercise, try splitting your workout into two short sessions. The first session of 15 to 20 minutes can be done before work or at lunchtime; the second, for another 15 to 20 minutes, can be squeezed in after work. In this scenario try to do short, but intensive, exercises.

A special note to smokers: A few of my patients quit smoking simply by starting the Carb Cycling Diet with exercise. In the beginning they tried to exercise to get in shape and continue to smoke, but later realized these two activities do not mix together well. Their mindsets changed and shifted towards protecting health via exercise and nutrition. As a result, they never picked up a cigarette again.

It is never too late to start exercising and adjusting your diet. Imagine a metaphoric finish line and your prizes: health and quality retirement years. The Carb Cycling Diet, combined with exercise, will protect you from diabetes, osteoarthritis, osteoporosis, cardiovascular diseases, and many forms of cancer. It will postpone aging and age-related metabolic decline. And all of these benefits come with just one hour of exercise three to five days a week and few restrictions on what you can eat.

The Carb Cycling Diet Schedule

Use this template to plan your meals and exercise on a week-by-week basis. Photocopy it and keep reusing it as necessary.

The CARB CYCLING DIET	MON	TUES	WED	THURS	FRI	SAT	SUN
GOAL							
DIET							
EXERCISE							
CARB INTAKE (in grams)							

Glossary

Aerobic exercise: Any physical activity performed at low to moderate intensity.

Amino acids: A product of the digestion of protein. Amino acids are the building blocks of protein.

Anaerobic exercise: any physical activity performed at high intensity, when energy need is extreme. In strength training it corresponds to weight that is more than 50% of 1-RM.

Anabolism: The part of metabolism that builds and restores tissues.

Anabolic hormones: The hormones that stimulate anabolism: Human Growth Hormone, growth factors, testosterone, insulin.

Basal Metabolic Rate (BMR): The number of calories necessary to maintain your body's basic functions at rest.

Carbohydrates: Sugars and starches that supply energy to the body. There are two kinds of carbohydrates: refined carbohydrates, like cakes and cookies, are the starches left when whole grains are highly refined through milling; unrefined carbohydrates are whole grains that are cracked or cut, not milled so they retain their fiber, like oatmeal, pearl barley, and brown rice. 1 gram of carbohydrate produces four calories when burned for energy.

Catabolism: The part of metabolism that breaks down tissues and leads to fat loss.

Catabolic hormones: The hormones that stimulate breaking down fat and protein: cortisol, epinephrine, glucagon, thyroid hormones.

Circuit training: A form of strength training exercise performed in a sequence.

Fat: The body stores fat as triglycerides (fatty acids and glycerol combined together) that are accumulated inside of fat cells. The more triglycerides fat cells accumulate the bigger they are. One gram of fat produces nine calories when used for energy.

Fatty acids: A building blocks of fats. It is the end product of dietary fat digestion.

Fructose: The type of sugar found in fruits and honey. Fructose does not trigger an insulin secretion as much as other sugars do.

Glucose: A simple sugar and the product of the digestion of carbohydrates. Glucose is a single sugar molecule (monosaccharide) related to table sugar (sucrose).

Glycogen: The storage form of glucose molecules.

Hormones: Chemical messengers that influence metabolic activities, cell division, and development.

Insulin: A hormone produced by the pancreas gland. This vital hormone controls the blood's glucose concentration.

Interval training: A form of training that consists of repetitions of exercise and intervals of relative rest. High Intensity Interval Training (HIIT) is a form of anaerobic training, when exercise is performed with high intensity that is 75 percent or more of maximum intensity.

Metabolism: A set of biochemical reactions that take place inside the body. Metabolism is the sum of all biochemical processes involved in life, the process by which energy is produced. Metabolism follows two pathways: catabolism (destroying) and anabolism (building).

Muscle: Muscles contain specific proteins that are responsible for contraction.

One-repetition maximum (1-RM): the amount of weight you can lift only once. Check it periodically, since when strength increases 1-RM increases too. Use weights that are more than 50 percent of your 1-RM on normal-carb days. Use weights that are less than 50 percent of 1-RM during circuit training.

Protein: Proteins are the main structural material of the body. They are important structural components of cells and tissues. They are made up of amino acids. Muscles contain large amounts of protein. Proteins produce four calories when burned for energy.

Repetition (rep): A number of times you repeat the move in each set.

Set: A group of consecutive repetitions performed without rest. For example, if you performed 10 push-ups 2 times with 1 minute rest in between it would be 2 sets of 10 reps.

Steroids: Lipid derivatives that have rings of carbon atoms. The most common steroid is cholesterol. Sex hormones, steroid hormones from adrenal gland, and vitamin D are all steroids and are derivatives of cholesterol.

Triglycerides: The major form of fat. The body stores fat as triglycerides.

Whey protein: "Whey" is the name given to the watery part of milk that remains after making cheese. Whey is, in fact, a natural byproduct of cheese manufacturing that is rich in lactose, essential amino acids, and minerals.

Resources and Suppliers

Food and Supplements Suppliers
CYCLING DIET
Most of the supplements can be ordered on www.CyclingDiet.com.

ARIZONA BEVERAGE CO.
5 Dakota Dr., Suite 205
Lake Success, NY 11042
1-800-TEA-3775 (1-800-832-3775)
www.arizonabev.com
Makers of Extreme Energy Shot, and other beverages.

BIOCHEM SPORTS AND FITNESS SYSTEMS
Country Life Vitamins
180 Vanderbilt Motor Parkway
Hauppauge, NY 11778
800-645-5768
www.biochem-fitness.com
Makers of Ultimate Carb Phaser 1000, and other sports supplements.

KNOX
www.kraftfoods.com/knox
Makers of NutraJoint Gelatine.

NATURE'S PLUS
(800)645-9500
www.naturesplus.com
Makers of Ultra Sugar Control and other energy supplements.

Now Foods

395 S. Glen Ellyn Road
Bloomingdale, IL 60108
www.nowfoods.com
Makers of vitamin B-50 and other vitamins, minerals, and herbs.

Universal Nutrition

3 Terminal Rd
New Brunswick, NJ 08901
800.872.0101
732.509.0458 (fax)
www.universalnutrition.com
Makers of CarniTech Liquid Carnitine Complex and other supplements.

Yamamotoyama

122 Voyager Street
Pomona, California 91768
909-594-7586
909-595-5849 (fax)
www.yamamotoyama.com
Makers of a Japanese green tea.

Sports Organizations and Resources

AMERICAN COLLEGE OF SPORTS MEDICINE

P.O. Box 1440

Indianapolis, IN 46206-1440

National Center (317) 637-9200

This 50-year-old organization has a web site, www.acsm.org. While part of the website is reserved for members of the ASCM, it does offer general health and fitness information. Under a tab for health and fitness information, you can calculate your maximum (theoretical) heart rate (based on your age) and from that determine your lower and upper limits of allowable heartbeat during high intensity exercise workouts. There is good advice about starting slowly and working up, along with a warning that the most dangerous choice is not to exercise at all.

AMERICAN VOLKSSPORT ASSOCIATION (AVA)

1001 Pat Brooker Road, Suite 101

Universal City, TX 78148

1-800-830-WALK

avahg@ava.org.

Volkssport is a German-derived term that embraces such sports as walking, swimming, skiing, snowshoeing, and biking.

THE BODY SCULPTING BIBLE SERIES BY JAMES VILLEPIGUE AND HUGO RIVERA

Hatherleigh Press

5-22 46th Avenue, Suite 200

Long Island City, NY 11101

As seen on *Live with Regis and Kelly* and *Good Day New York* and in *Fitness, Women's World, Oxygen, Modern Bride, Newsday, Boston Globe, Miami Herald, Houston Chronicle, Women's Health and Fitness, Musclemag International*, and many more, this bestselling series of weight-training book offers cutting-edge workouts for men and women to achieve their perfect bodies in less time.

COOL RUNNING

Cool Sports, Inc.

PO Box 299

Londonderry, NH, 03053

603-845-0190 ext: 6

Cool Running sponsors the website www.CoolRunning.com. They offer news about amateur and Olympic racing. They also offer training programs for new and experienced runners. New runners can click the Training tab and get useful subdirectories offering tips and advice, performance, new runner signup, training schedules, and online coaching.

GETFITNOW.COM

www.GetFitNow.com

This website is a powerful resource for anyone seeking fitness advice, news, discussion forums, and more.

Bibliography

Abe, T., Kawakami, Y., Sugita, M., & Fukunaga, T. (1997). "Relationship between Training Frequency and Subcutaneous and Visceral Fat in Women," *Medicine and Science in Sports and Exercise,* 29:1549–1553.

Armstrong, Lawrence E. (2002). "Caffeine, Body Fluid-Electrolyte Balance, and Exercise Performance," *International Journal of Sport Nutrition and Exercise Metabolism,* 12:2:189–206.

Baba, N. Hwalla, Sawaya, S., Torbay, N., Habbal, Z., Azar, S., and Hashim, S.A. (1999). "High Protein vs. High Carbohydrate Hypoenergetic Diet for the Treatment of Obese Hyperinsulinemic subjects." *International Journal of Obesity,* 23:11:1202–1206.

Bahrke, M.S., and Yessalis, C.E. (2002). *Performance–Enhancing Substances in Sport and Exercise.* Champaign, IL: Human Kinetics.

Below, P.R., Mora-Rodriguez, J., and Coyle, E.F. (1995). "Fluid and Carbohydrate Ingestion Independently Improve Performance During 1 hour of Intense Exercise," *Medicine and Science in Sports and Exercise* 27:200–210.

Bergstorm, J.L., Hermansen, Hultman, E., and Saltin, B. (1967). "Diet, Muscle Glycogen and Physical Performance," *Acta Physiologica* Scandinavica, 71:140–150.

Biolo, G., Declan Fleming , R.Y., and Wolfe, R.R. (1995). "Physiologic Hyperinsulinemia Stimulates Protein Synthesis and Enhances Transport of Selected Amino Acids in Human Skeletal Muscle," *The Journal of Clinical Investigation,* 95:811–819.

Browell, K.D., Steen, S.N., and Wilmore, J.R. (1990). "Weight Regulation Practices in Athletes: Analysis of Metabolic and Health Effects," *Medicine & Science in Sports & Exercise,* 19:546–556.

Buemann, B., & Tremblay, A. (1996). "Effects of Exercise Training on Abdominal Obesity and Related Metabolic Complications," *Sports Medicine,* 21:191–212.

Bullough, C.R., Gilette, C.A., Harris, M.A., and Melby, C.L. (1995). "Interaction of Acute Changes in Exercise Energy Expenditure and Energy Intake on Resting Metabolic Rate," *American Journal of Clinical Nutrition,* 61:473–481.

Consitt, L.A., Copeland, J.L., and Tremblay, J.S. (2001). "Hormone Responses to Resistance vs. Endurance Exercise in Premenopausal Females," *Canadian Journal of Applied Physiology,* 26:6.

Costill D.L., Sherman, W.M., and Fink, W.J. (1981). "The Role of Dietary Carbohydrate in Muscle Glycogen Resynthesis after Strenuous Running," *American Journal of Clinical Nutrition,* 34:1831–1836.

Flynn, M.G., Costill, D.L., Kirwan, J.P., Mitchell, J.B., and Hounmard, J.A. (1990). "Fat Storage in Athletes: Metabolic and Hormonal Responses to Swimming and Running," *International Journal of Sports Medicine,* 11:433–440.

Fried, K.E., Moore, R.J., Hoyt, R.W., Marchitelli, L.J., Martinez-Lopez, L.E., and Askew, E.W. (2000). "Endocrine Markers of Semis-tarvation in Healthy Lean Men in a Multistressor Environment," *Journal of Applied Physiology,* 88:5:1820–1830.

Hackney, A.C., Szczepanowska, E., and Viru, A.M. (2003). "Basal Testicular Testosterone Production in Endurance-Trained Men Is Suppressed," *European Journal of Applied Physiology, 89:198–201.*

Hakkinen, K., Kraemer, W.J., Pakarinen, A., Triplett-McBride, T. McBride, J.M., Hakkinen, A., Alen, J., McGuigan, M.R., Bronks, R., and Newton, R.U. (2002). "Effects of Heavy Resistance/Power Training on Maximal Strength, Muscle Morphology, and Hor-monal Response Patterns in 60- to 75-Year-Old Men and Women," *Canadian Journal of Applied Physiology,* 27:3.

Heiss, C.J., Sanborn, C.F., Nichols, D.L. (1995). "Associations of Body Fat Distribution, Circulating Sex Hormones, and Bone Den-sity in Postmenopausal Women," *Journal of Clinical Endocrinology,* 80:1591–1596.

Henriksen, E.J. (2002). "Exercise Effects of Muscle Insulin Sig-naling and Action Invited Review: Effects of Acute Exercise and Exercise Training on Insulin Resistance," *Journal of Applied Physiol-ogy,* 93:788–796.

Ivy, J.L., Lee, M.C., and Reed, M.J. (1988). "Muscle Glycogen Storage after Different Amounts of Carbohydrate Ingestion," *Journal of Applied Physiology,* 65:20018–20023.

Jacks, D.E., Sowash, J., Anning, J., McGloughlin, T., and Andres, F. (2002). "Effect of Exercise at Three Exercise Intensities on Salivary Cortisol," *Journal of Strength and Conditioning Research* 16:286–289.

Kimball, S.R., Farrell, P.A., and Jefferson, L.S. (2002). "Exercise Effects on Muscle Insulin Signaling and Action Invited Review: Role of Insulin in Translational Control of Protein Synthesis in Skeletal Muscle by Amino Acids or Exercise," *Journal of Applied Physiology,* 93:1168–1180.

Kircher M.A., Samojlik, E., Drejka, M. (1991). "Sex Hormone Metabolism in Upper and Lower Body Obesity," *International Journal of Obesity,* 15:101–108.

Kirwan, J.P., O'Gorman, D., and Evans, W.J. (1988). "A Moderate Glycemic Meal before Endurance Exercise Can Enhance Performance," *Journal of Applied Physiology,* 84:1:53–59.

Kissebah, A.H., Evans D.J, and Wilson, C.R. (1985). *Endocrine Characteristics in Regional Obesities: Role of Sex Steroids,* San Diego: Elsevier Science.

Koceja, D.M., and Hamilton, E.J. (1997). "A Meta Analysis of the Past 25 Years of Weight Loss Research Using Diet, Exercise, or Diet Plus Exercise Intervention," *International Journal of Obesity,* 21:941–947.

Kokkoris, P., Pi-Sunyer, F.X. (2003). "Obesity and Endocrine Disease," *Endocrinology and Metabolism Clinics of North America.* 32:4:895–914.

Kraemer, W.J., Volek, J.S., Clark, K.L., Gordon, S.E., Puhl, S.M., Koziris, L.P., McBride, J.M., Triplett-McBride, N.T., Putukian, M., Newton, R.U., Hakkinen, K., Bush, J.A., and Sebastianelli, W.J. (1999). "Influence of Exercise Training on Physiological and Performance Changes with Weight Loss in Men," *Medicine and Science in Sports and Exercise,* 31:1320–1329.

Mulligan, K., and Butterfield, G.E. (1990). "Discrepancies between Energy Intake and Expenditure in Physically Active Women," *British Journal of Nutrition,* 64:23–36.

Nind, B.C. and Kraemer, W.J. (2001). "Testosterone Responses after Resistance Exercise in Women: Influence of Regional Fat Distribution," *International Journal of Sport Nutrition and Exercise Metabolism,* 11:4:451–465.

Nind, B.C. Hymer, W.C., Deaver, D.R., and Kraemer, W.J. (2001). "Growth Hormone Pulsatility Profile Characteristics Following Acute Heavy Resistance Exercise," *Journal of Applied Physiology,* Jul:91(1):163–72.

Nind, B.C., Harman, E.A., Marx, J.O., Gotshalk, L.A., Frykman, P.N., Lammi, E., Palmer, C., and Kraemer, W.J. (2000). "Regional Body Composition Changes in Women after 6 Months of Periodized Physical Training," *Journal of Applied Physiology,* 88:2251–2259.

Pederson, S.B. Borglum, J.D., and Brixen, K. (1995). "Relationship between Sex Hormones, Body Composition and Metabolic Risk Parameters in Premenopausal Women," *European Journal of Endocrinology,* 133:200–206.

Radak, Z. (2002). *Free Radicals in Exercise and Aging,* Champaign, IL: Human Kinetics.

Ross, R., Dagnone, D., Jones, P.J.H., Smith, H., Paddags, A., Hudson, R., and Janssen, I. (2000). "Reduction in Obesity and Related Comorbid Conditions after Diet-Induced Weight Loss or Exercise-Induced Weight Loss in Men," *Annals of Internal Medicine,* 133:92–103.

Rudman, D., Feller, A.G., Nagraj, H.S., Gergans, G.A., Lalitha, P.Y., Goldberg, A.F., Schlenker, R.A., Cohn, L., Rudman, I.W., and Mattson, D.E. (1990). "Effects of Human Growth Hormone in Men over 60 Years Old," *New England Journal of Medicine,* 323:1.

Salway, J.G. (2000). *Metabolism at a Glance,* London: Blackwell Science.

Saris, W.M., Astrup, A., Prentice, A.M., Zunft, H.F., Formiguera, X., Raben, A., Poppitt, S.D., Seppelt, B., Johnston, S., Vasilaras, T.H., and Keogh, G.F. (2000). "Randomized Controlled Trial of Changes in Dietary Carbohydrate–Fat Ratio and Simple vs. Complex Carbohydrates on Body Weight and Blood Lipids: The CARMEN Study," *International Journal of Obesity,* 24:10:1310–1318.

Stokes, K.A., Nevill, M.E., Hall, G.M., and Lakomy, H.K.A. (2002). "Growth Hormone Responses to Repeated Maximal Cycle Ergometer Exercise at Different Pedaling Rates," *Journal of Applied Physiology,* 92:2:602–608.

Siff, M. C., and Verkhoshansky, Y.V. (1999). *Supertraining. Colorado: Everything Track and Field.*

Tipton, K.D. (2001). "Muscle Protein Metabolism in The Elderly: Influence of Exercise and Nutrition," *Canadian Journal of Applied Physiology*, 26:6.

Tsai, E.C., Boyko, E.J., Leonetti, D.L., and Fujimoto, W.Y. (2000). "Low Serum Testosterone Level as a Predictor of Increased Visceral Fat in Japanese-American Men," *International Journal of Obesity and Related Metabolic Disorders*, 24:485–491.

Utter, A.C., Nieman, D.C., Shannonhouse, E.M., Butterworth, D.E., and Nieman, C.N. (1998). "Influence of Diet and/or Exercise on Body Composition and Cardio-Respiratory Fitness in Obese Women," *International Journal of Sport Nutrition*, 8:213–222.

Van Aggel-Leijssen, D.P.C., Saris, W.H.M., Hul, G.B., & van Baak, M.A. (2001). "Short-Term Effects of Weight Loss with or without Low-Intensity Exercise Training on Fat Metabolism in Obese Men," *American Journal of Clinical Nutrition, 73:523–531*.

Index

7-Keto, 192–193, 197

A

adapting the carb cycling diet,
206–207

adaptive heat generation, 25

adipose tissue, 29

adjusting the diet to your life,
68–69

adrenal glands, 27

advanced exercise program, 148

aerobic exercise, 15, 130, 215

aerobic versus anaerobic exercise,
129

after exercise dessert, 123

age, effects of, 32–433, 46, 144,
145, 206

alcohol consumption, 71

Alpha Lipoic acid, 153, 197, 198

American Dietary Association, 38

amino acids, 215

anabolic hormones, 13, 14, 22, 23,
27, 45–46, 127, 215

anabolism, 15, 23, 24, 25, 28, 31,
46, 58, 60, 129, 215

anaerobic exercise, 130–1321, 215

anaerobic weight lifting, 15

assisted dips, 167

Atkins Diet, 16

ATP, 48, 49

B

baked salmon, 118

barbell press, 163

basal metabolic rate (BMR), 25,
26, 42, 132, 142, 215

bean salad, 112

beans, consumption of, 77

beef stroganoff, 118

beginner exercise program, 147

bench dips, 168

benefits of carb cycling, 39–40

bent-over raises, 162

blood sugar stabilizer, as a, 196

Body Sculpting Bible, 155

bone loss, 39

Boswellia extract, 153, 199

branched-chain amino acids
(BCAA), 44, 196

breakfast yogurt fruit smoothie,
110

brown and wild rice eggplant
salad, 99

Bulgarian cold cucumber soup in
yogurt, 103

bulking cycles, 181

C

C-Reactive protein, 75

caffeine, 194

calcium, 39, 153, 183, 198
calorie balance, 24
calorie cycling, 61
calorie restricted diets
    consequences of, 38–39
    depression, 38
    deprivation diets, downfalls of,
        36–39
    disadvantages of, 35–36
    hair loss, 38
    immune system, weakening of
        the, 38
    joint pain, 38
    libido, lack of, 38
    malnutrition, 37
    muscle loss, 39
    osteoporosis, 39
    overtraining, 36
    self-destroying catabolic mode,
        37
    slow metabolism (diminished
        BMR), 38
    undernutrition, 37
    wrinkles, 38
calories, 15, 24, 59–62
cancer, protection against, 128
carb cycling regimens, 57–58
carbohydrates, 47, 51–52, 215
CarniTech Liquid Carnitine
    Complex, 197
catabolic hormones, 23, 216
catabolism, 15, 23, 24, 25, 28, 31,

58, 129, 215
change of pace, incorporating a,
    140–141
chicken and bean burrito, 101
chicken, feta cheese, and spinach
    salad, 112
chocolate fudge dessert
chondroitin sulfate, 153, 199
chromium, 196
chronic disease, protection
    against, 128
circuit training, 132–133,
    135–136, 216
    assisted dips, 167
    barbell press, 163
    bench dips, 168
    bent-over raises, 162
    dumbbell bench press, 156
    dumbbell extensions, 166
    dumbbell flyes, 157
    dumbbell squat, 173
    floor crunches, 169
    incline dumbbell curl, 164
    leg extension, 171
    leg press, 172
    lower body and ab exercises,
        155
    one-arm dumbbell rows, 159
    push ups, 158
    role of, 154
    seated dumbbell curl, 165
    side raises, 160

upper body weight lifting
exercises, 154

V-up, 170

wide grip pulldowns, 160

Coenzyme Q-10, 28, 130, 153,
195, 197

completing the six-week carb
cycling program, 72–73

connective tissue proteins, 43

cortisol, 23, 27

cravings, 96, 197

creole shrimp stew, 115

cucumber tomato salad in sour
cream sauce, 105

cutting cycles, 181

D

daily calorie needs, 24, 26, 31, 61,
206

depression, 38

deprivation diets, downfalls of,
36–39

DHEA, 13, 14, 138, 190, 192

diet pills, 196

diet schedule, 213

digestion of food, 25, 26

DMAE (dimethylaminoethanol),
195, 197

dumbbell bench press, 156

dumbbell extensions, 166

dumbbell flyes, 157

dumbbell squat, 173

E

eggplant salad, 105

eggplant sandwich, 100

energy during exercise,
maintaining, 143

energy reserve, 30

energy-increasing supplements,
194–196, 197

estrogen, 26, 27

exercise

advanced exercise program,
148

aerobic exercise, 130

aerobic versus anaerobic
exercise, 129

age, effects of, 144, 145

anabolic hormones, 127

anaerobic exercise,
130–132

beginner exercise program,
147

benefits of, 127–128

boosting anabolic hormones
through, 45–46

cancer, protection against, 128

carb cycling diet, and the,
136–138

carbohydrate restriction, and,
140

change of pace, incorporating
a, 140–141

chronic disease, protection
　　against, 128
circuit training, 132–133,
　　135–136 (See Circuit
　　training)
energy during exercise,
　　maintaining, 143
guidelines, 151–152
high-intensity workouts,
　　138–140
Human Growth Hormone
　　(HGH), 127
intermediate exercise program,
　　148
interval training, 132–134,
　　133, 141, 174–176
joint degeneration, 152, 153
losing weight without, 62–63
metabolism, increasing your,
　　178
muscle soreness, 153
nutritional supplementation,
　　153
plateau, breaking the, 176–177
program 1 for men, 150
program 1 for women, 150
risks associated with vigorous
　　exercise, 143–145
role of, 25
slow-fast training, 133, 134,
　　176
taking a break from exercise,
　　141–142
weight lifting for women, 142
Extreme Energy Shot, 143, 198

F

false hunger, 67
fat, 31, 216
fat cells bank, 29
fat deposition, 15, 21, 23, 43–45,
　　49
fat loss stages, 58–59
fatty acids, essential, 153, 216
feta cheese scrambled eggs, 111
floor crunches, 169
free radicals, 46
French onion soup low-carb
　　style, 104
fructose, 216

G

gelatine, 198
glucagon, 23, 27
glucosamine, 153, 199
glucose, 29, 216
glucose metabolism, 26
glucose uptake, 28–29
glycemic index, 49, 50–51
glycogen, 27, 30, 43, 62, 131, 135,
　　138, 216
glycogen molecule, 29–30
green tea, 77, 197
guarana seeds, 194–195

H

hair loss, 38
hara hachi-bu, 68, 69
Healthy Breakfast, 45, 65, 75, 108
heart rate monitor, 154
HGH secretagoges, 191–192
high-intensity workouts, 138–140
hormonal replacement therapy, 13
hormones, role of, 26–27, 216
Human Growth Hormone
    (HGH), 13, 23, 26, 27, 127,
    138, 189, 190–191
hyaluronic acid, 153, 199
Hydroxycut, 196

I

immune system, weakening of
    the, 38
incline dumbbell curl, 164
insulin, 21, 28–29, 29, 216
insulin receptors, 51
intermediate exercise program,
    148
interval training, 132–134, 133,
    141, 174–176, 217
iodine, 27

J

joint degeneration, 152, 153
joint pain, 38
joint recovery after exercise, 198

K

kelp, 28, 194, 198
kilocalories, 15

L

L-arginine, 191
L-carnitine, 96, 197
L-tyrosine, 28, 193–194
Lecithin, 153
Lecithin softgels, 198
leg extension, 171
leg press, 172
Level A, 59
Level B, 59
Level C, 59, 69
libido, lack of, 38
lifestyle changes, making, 22
limited-carb days, 15, 69, 70, 204
    Level A meal plans, 81–85
    Level B meal plans, 86–90
    Level C meal plans, 91–95
    meal plans, 80–96
    recipes (See Recipes)
liver bank, 29
liver glycogen, 44, 45, 62
losing fat, 31
lower body and ab exercises, 155

M

macrocycling, 182, 183, 184
malnutrition, 37

maltodextrin, 67

managing the carb cycling diet, 67–68

marinated aromatized lamb kabobs, 107

MAX effort exercise, 32, 134, 139, 145, 178–179

melatonin, 193

metabolic decline, 22

metabolic rate, 27

metabolism, 15, 22–24, 25–26, 26, 206, 217

   aging, and, 32–433

   boosters, 190

   increasing your, 178

   preventing slowdown, 41–42

mitochondria, 28

monosaccharide, 29

mozzerella sandwich, 100

MSM, 153, 199

multivitamin, use of, 38

muscle, 217

muscle bank, 29

muscle glycogen, 62

muscle loss, 39

muscle protein, 43

muscle soreness, 153

mushroom and cheese scrambled eggs, 110

myofibrils, 139

N

NADH (Nictinamide Adenine Dinucleotide), 130, 195–196, 198

negative calorie balance, 24, 31, 65, 129

New England Clam Chowder, 98

normal-carb days, 15, 69, 181, 203

   meal plans, 76–80

Nutrajoint, 198

nutritional supplementation, 153

O

Omega-3, 198

Omega-6, 198

Omega-9, 198

one-arm dumbbell rows, 159

one-repetition maximum, 217

osteoporosis, 39, 142

overtraining, 36

overweight or obese, for the, 199

P

pancreas, 21, 28

physical activity, 25, 26

plateau, breaking the, 176–177

poached American summer salmon, 119

pork chops with vegetable mix, 120

positive calorie balance, 31, 46, 76, 129, 139, 206

post-exercise supplements, 198

pre-exercise morning supplements, 197–198

protein, 217

protein synthesis, 29

protein, building, 31, 32

protein, preventing loss of, 42–43

push ups, 158

Q

quick family salsa, 122

R

rebound hunger, 67

recipes

    after exercise dessert, 123

    baked salmon, 118

    bean salad, 112

    beef stroganoff, 118

    breakfast yogurt fruit smoothie, 110

    brown and wild rice eggplant salad, 99

    Bulgarian cold cucumber soup in yogurt, 103

    chicken and bean burrito, 101

    chicken, feta cheese, and spinach salad, 112

    chocolate fudge dessert

    creole shrimp stew, 115

    cucumber tomato salad in sour cream sauce, 105

    eggplant salad, 105

    eggplant sandwich, 100

    feta cheese scrambled eggs, 111

    French onion soup low-carb style, 104

    Healthy Breakfast, 108

    marinated aromatized lamb kabobs, 107

    mozzerella sandwich, 100

    mushroom and cheese scrambled eggs, 110

    New England Clam Chowder, 98

    poached American summer salmon, 119

    pork chops with vegetable mix, 120

    quick family salsa, 122

    roast chicken with potatoes, 102

    sautéed chicken with arti choke hearts and onions, 117

    scallop and shrimp salad, 113

    seafood salad, 114

    Spanish style chicken, 116

    spinach and cheese omelette, 111

    strawberry smoothie, 109

stuffed tri-color peppers, 121
Sunday morning breakfast, 108
tasty low-fat tuna sandwich, 106
whey protein shake, 109
refined carbohydrates, 15, 22,
    39, 40–41, 47, 48, 202
regimens, 57–59
    program 1 for men, 64
    program 1 for women, 64
    program 2 for men, 66
    program 2 for women, 66
repetition, 217
rest days, 36
roast chicken with potatoes, 102

S

sautéed chicken with artichoke
    hearts and onions, 117
scallop and shrimp salad, 113
sea cucumber, 153, 199
seafood salad, 114
seated dumbbell curl, 165
self-destroying catabolic mode, 37
set, 218
sex hormones, 190
side raises, 160
slow metabolism (diminished
    BMR), 38
slow-fast training, 133, 134, 176
soda, consumption of, 67
South Beach Diet, 16
Spanish style chicken, 116

spinach and cheese omelette, 111
Splenda, 177
sports drinks, 143
starve and binge, 82
steroids, 218
Stevia Plus, 177
strawberry smoothie, 109
stuffed tri-color peppers, 121
sugar control supplements, 96
sugar, role of, 40–41
Sunday morning breakfast, 108
supplements
    7-Keto, 192–193, 197
    blood sugar stabilizer, as a, 196
    caffeine, 194
    calcium, 39, 153, 183, 198
    Coenzyme Q-10, 28, 130,
        153, 195, 197
    craving for sweets, to relieve,
        197
    DHEA, 13, 14, 138, 190, 192
    diet pills, 196
    DMAE (dimethy-
        laminoethanol), 195, 197
    energy-increasing
        supplements, 194–196, 197
    guarana seeds, 194–195
    HGH secretagoges, 191–192
    Human Growth Hormone
        (HGH), 13, 23, 26, 27,
        127, 138, 189, 190–191
    joint recovery after exercise,

198
kelp, 28, 198
kelp for iodine, 194
L-arginine, 191
L-carnitine, 96, 197
L-tyrosine, 28, 193–194
limited-carb days, on, 198
melatonin, 193
metabolism boosters, 190
NADH (Nictinamide Adenine
    Dinucleotide), 195–196,
    198
overweight or obese, for the,
    199
post-exercise supplements, 198
pre-exercise morning
    supplements, 197–198
sex hormones, 190
snack, as a, 196
thyroid hormone, 193
use of, 46, 75, 153, 189–190,
    196–197
Vitamin B-complex, 197

T

tasty low-fat tuna sandwichh, 106
temperature control, 26
testosterone, 13, 23, 26, 27, 138,
    142
Thermo Gain, 196
thyroid hormone, 27, 28, 193
thyroxine, 27

triglycerides (TG), 29, 218
type 2 diabetes, 22
tyrosine, 27

U

Ultimate Carb Phaser 1000, 197
Ultra Sugar Control, 197
undernutrition, 37
unrefined carbohydrates, 47, 48
upper body weight lifting exer-
    cises, 154

V

V-up, 170
vanadium, 196
Vitamin B-50, 197
Vitamin B-complex, 197
Vitamin C, 153, 198
Vitamin E, 153, 198

W

weight lifting for women, 142
weight training, 46, 131, 205
whey protein, 44, 65, 96, 196,
    198, 218
whey protein shake, 109
wide grip pulldowns, 160
wrinkles, 38

X

Xenadrine, 196

About the Author

Dr. Roman Malkov, graduated from Moscow Medical University in 1989 as a gastroenterologist. For several years, he served as the Attending Physician at Central Hospital in Moscow and as a Nutritional Consultant for the Russian National Rowing Team. In 1997, he passed the U.S. Medical License examination. He is an Alliance member of the American College of Sports Medicine. His private practice is established in New York City where he is a consultant to professional athletes and fitness enthusiasts. Founder and president of Nutrigen International, Inc., he also practices sports nutrition and nutrigenomics.